Vegetarian
Post Liver Transplant Recipes

Offers Nutrient-Packed Delicious Breakfast, Lunch, Dinner, Snacks and Smoothie Options to Promote Smooth Recovery.

By
CYNTHIA LEONARD

TABLE OF CONTENTS

TABLE OF CONTENTS   2

INTRODUCTION   9

ABOUT THIS RECIPE BOOK   9

BREAKFAST MEALS   12

Quinoa Breakfast Bowl   12

Avocado Toast with Spinach and Tomato   14

Vegetable Omelette with Herbs   16

Chia Seed Pudding with Berries   18

Greek Yoghurt Parfait with·Granola   20

Banana Walnut Muffins   22

Spinach and Mushroom Frittata   24

Overnight Oats with Almond Milk and Fruits   26

Tofu Scramble with Peppers and Onions   28

Vegan Breakfast Burrito   30

Buckwheat Pancakes with Maple Syrup   32

Fruit Smoothie Bowl with Nut Butter   34

Zucchini and Carrot Fritters   36

Breakfast Quiche with Sun-Dried Tomatoes   37

Veggie Breakfast Wrap with Hummus   39

LUNCH MEALS   42

Lentil Soup with Vegetables   42

Quinoa Salad with Roasted Vegetables   44

Chickpea Salad with Lemon-Tahini Dressing 46

Caprese Salad with Balsamic Glaze 48

Vegetable Stir-Fry with Tofu 49

Sweet Potato and Black Bean Quesadillas 52

Greek Salad with Tzatziki Dressing 55

Spinach and Feta Stuffed Bell Peppers 57

Mushroom Barley Risotto 59

Eggplant Parmesan with Marinara Sauce 61

Cauliflower Fried Rice 65

Falafel Wraps with Hummus and Veggies 67

Tomato Basil Bruschetta 70

Quinoa and Black Bean Stuffed Peppers 72

Veggie Sushi Rolls with Soy Sauce 74

DINNER MEALS

DINNER MEALS 78

Butternut Squash Soup with Croutons 78

Ratatouille with Herbed Couscous 81

Vegetable Lasagna with Cashew Cheese 83

Stuffed Portobello Mushrooms with Quinoa and Spinach 86

Thai Green Curry with Tofu and Vegetables 88

Eggplant and Chickpea Tagine 91

Spinach and Ricotta Stuffed Shells 93

Cauliflower Steak with Chimichurri Sauce 96

Black Bean and Corn Enchiladas 98

Veggie Stir-Fry Noodles 102

Creamy Mushroom Risotto 104

Spinach and Artichoke Stuffed Spaghetti Squash 106

Lentil Shepherd's Pie 109

Veggie Tikka Masala with Basmati Rice 112

Grilled Vegetable Skewers with Quinoa Pilaf 115

SNACKS OPTIONS 118

Hummus and Veggie Sticks 118

Trail Mix with Nuts and Dried Fruits 120

Baked Kale Chips 122

Avocado Slices on Whole Grain Crackers 124

Apple Slices with Peanut Butter 125

Roasted Chickpeas with Spices 127

Rice Cakes with Almond Butter 129

Cucumber Slices with Cream Cheese and Dill 130

Guacamole with Baked Tortilla Chips 132

Energy Balls with Dates and Nuts 135

SMOOTHIE OPTIONS 138

Green Smoothie with Spinach, Banana and Almond Milk 138

Berry Blast Smoothie with Mixed Berries and Greek Yoghurt 139

Tropical Paradise Smoothie with Mango, Pineapple and
Coconut Milk 141

Chocolate Peanut Butter Smoothie with Protein Powder 142

Beetroot and Berry Smoothie with Flax Seeds 144

Cucumber Mint Cooler 146

Watermelon Basil Refresher 147

Golden Milk with Turmeric and Ginger 149

Pineapple Ginger Lemonade   151

Kiwi and Kale Smoothie   153

Carrot Orange Ginger Juice   154

Chia Seed Lemonade   156

INTRODUCTION

ABOUT THIS RECIPE BOOK

After a liver transplant, recovery is a crucial stage on the road to better health and wellbeing for the patient. Eating well is important for promoting the body's healing process, but **Vegans** may find it difficult to locate meals that are appropriate for after a transplant.

On the other hand - adopting a plant-based, vegetarian diet may provide a caring and nutritious strategy for recuperating after a transplant.

Plant-based diets have been increasingly recognised in recent years for their ability to support general health and facilitate recovery following a variety of medical operations, including liver transplantation. Vegetarian post-transplant dishes, with their emphasis on complete foods like fruits, vegetables, grains, legumes, nuts and seeds, provide vital vitamins, minerals, antioxidants and phytonutrients that are needed for healing and preserving good health.

A vegetarian diet may be especially beneficial for vegans who are having liver transplant surgery. Plant-based diets are low in cholesterol and saturated fats, which may help lower the risk of problems like obesity and cardiovascular disease, both of which can affect the transplant's long-term effectiveness.

Also, immune system support, gastrointestinal pain and inflammation are frequent postoperative issues that may be managed with the help of vegetarian post-transplant dishes.

A more seamless recuperation process may result from combining anti-inflammatory components like turmeric, ginger and leafy greens with meals high in fibre to support digestive health.

We will look at a range of tasty, high-nutrient vegetarian meals in this book, all of which are designed to satisfy the special dietary requirements of people who have had liver transplant surgery and yet maintain a vegan diet. These dishes, which range from filling grain bowls and salads loaded with protein to soothing soups and healthy smoothies are intended to satisfy the palate, provide vital nutrients and enhance general health.

These vegetarian recipes offer a tasty and nutritious way to support your journey towards optimal health and renewed vitality following liver transplant surgery, regardless of whether you're a vegan navigating the difficulties of post-transplant recovery or just looking to include more plant-based meals in your diet.

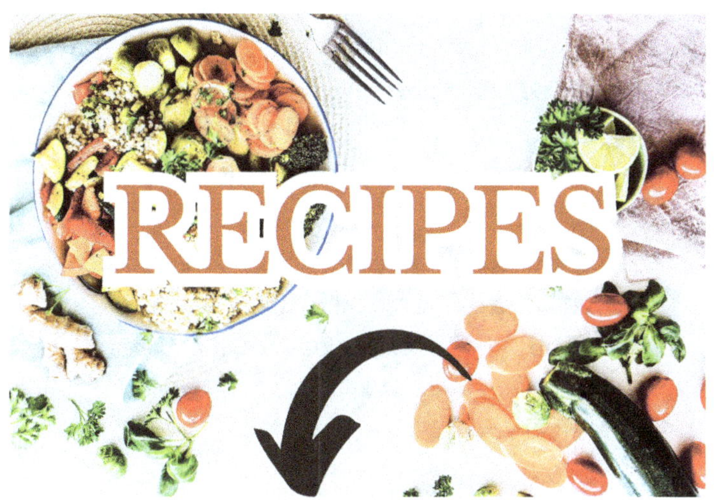

BREAKFAST MEALS

Quinoa Breakfast Bowl

Ingredients:

- One cup of rinsed quinoa
- two cups of water or veggie broth
- One tablespoon of olive or coconut oil
- One small onion, cut finely
- 2 minced garlic cloves
- 1 diced bell pepper
- 1 cup of chopped spinach or greens
- Salt and pepper.
- Avocado slices, cherry tomatoes, chopped cilantro, sliced almonds, crumbled feta cheese, fried or poached eggs are examples of *optional toppings*.

Instruction:

Quinoa should be combined with water or vegetable broth in a medium pot. After bringing to a boil, lower heat to a simmer, cover and cook for 15 to 20 minutes or until quinoa is tender and the water has been absorbed.

Using a fork, fluff the quinoa and put it aside.

Olive or coconut oil should be heated over medium heat in a big skillet.

Cook the chopped onion for 3–4 minutes or until it becomes transparent. Once aromatic, add the minced garlic and simmer for an additional minute.

Cook the chopped bell pepper in the pan for 2 to 3 minutes or until it starts to soften then add the chopped kale or spinach and simmer for a further 2 to 3 minutes or until wilted.

Add the cooked quinoa and continue to stir, combining everything well. To taste, add salt and pepper for seasoning.

Spoon the quinoa mixture into individual serving dishes.

Add any preferred toppings to each bowl, such as sliced avocado, chopped cilantro, cherry tomatoes, sliced almonds, crumbled feta cheese or fried or poached eggs.

Enjoy your quinoa breakfast bowl, which is both tasty and healthful, right away.

You are welcome to alter this recipe to suit your tastes by substituting other veggies, herbs or sources of protein.

Avocado Toast with Spinach and Tomato

Ingredients:

- 2 ripe avocados
- Four pieces of whole grain bread, or any other kind of bread
- One cup of newly harvested spinach
- One big tomato, cut into slices
- Salt and pepper.
- Flakes of red pepper *(optional)*
- Juice from lemons *(optional)*

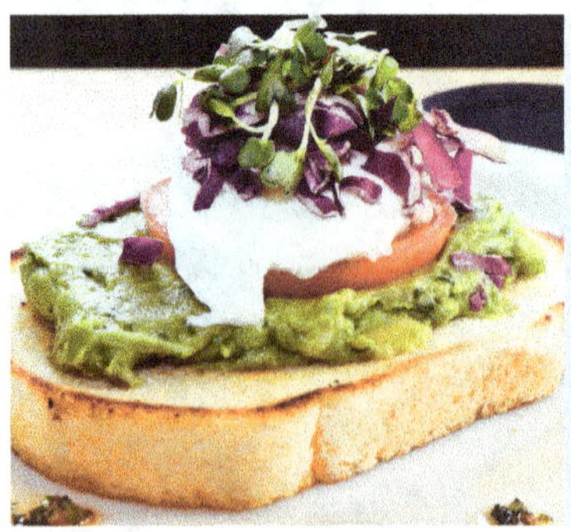 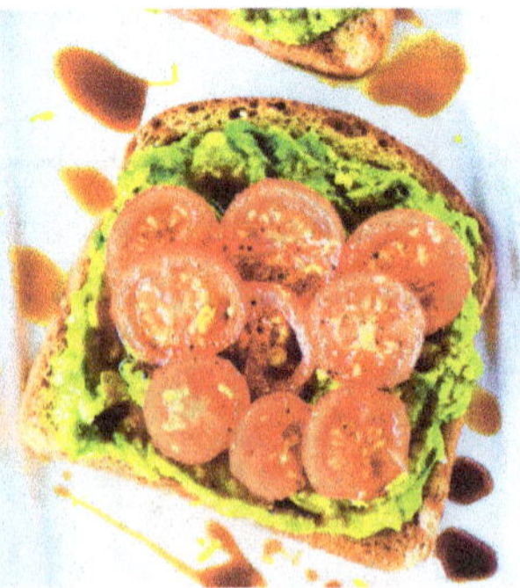

Instruction:

Toast the bread pieces first until they are crispy and golden brown with a little amount of olive oil in a pan over medium heat.

Prepare the avocados while the bread is toasting.
Halve them, remove the pits and transfer the meat to a basin. Using a fork, mash the avocado until the appropriate consistency is achieved.

If you would want to keep the avocado from browning, you may squeeze in a little lemon juice.

After toasting the bread, equally distribute the mashed avocado over each piece.

Arrange the baby spinach leaves over the avocado mixture.

Arrange tomato slices over the spinach.

If preferred, add some red pepper flakes, salt and pepper to the avocado toast.

Serve your tasty avocado toast with tomato and spinach right away.

Vegetable Omelette with Herbs

Ingredients:

- 3 eggs
- 1/4 cup of finely sliced bell peppers, any hue
- 1/4 cup of finely chopped onions
- 1/4 cup of tomatoes, chopped
- 1/4 cup of finely chopped spinach
- One tablespoon of finely chopped fresh herbs - such basil, chives or parsley
- Salt and pepper.
- One tablespoon of butter or olive oil
- Shredded cheese *(feta or cheddar)* is **optional.**

Instruction:

Beat the eggs together in a bowl until well mixed. Adjust the amount of salt and pepper to suit your taste.

In a nonstick skillet, preheat the butter or olive oil over medium heat.

To the skillet, add the chopped onions and bell peppers.
They should soften after 2 to 3 minutes of sautéing.

Then add the chopped tomatoes and spinach. Cook until the
spinach begins to wilt, about one to 2 more minutes.

Over the veggies in the pan, pour the beaten eggs. Allow the
eggs to cook without stirring for one minute.

Over the eggs, scatter the finely chopped fresh herbs. Add
some cheese to the eggs as well, if using.

To allow the raw eggs to flow to the edges, tilt the pan and
gently raise the omelette's edges with a spatula.

Gently fold one side of the omelette over the other to create
a half-moon shape after the eggs are nearly set but still a
little runny on top.

Cook the omelette for a further 1 to 2 minutes or until the
eggs are set and the cheese, *if used,* has melted.

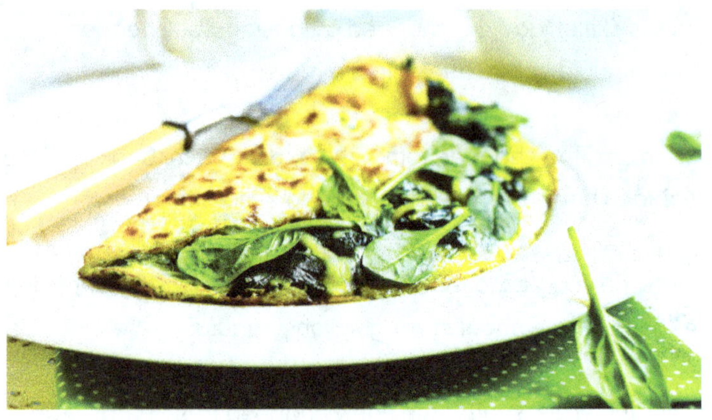

Transfer the omelette to a plate and Serve it warm.

Depending on your tastes, you may alter this recipe by adding or removing certain veggies or herbs.

Chia Seed Pudding with Berries

Ingredients:

- One-fourth cup chia seeds
- One cup almond milk, or any other kind of milk you like
- One tablespoon of maple syrup or honey, adjusted to taste
- Half a teaspoon of extract from vanilla
- ½ cup of mixed berries, including raspberries, blueberries, and strawberries

- Extra berries *(optional)* to garnish
- **Optional toppings** include shredded coconut or sliced almonds.

Instruction:

Combine the chia seeds, almond milk, honey/maple syrup and vanilla essence in a jar or dish. Mix well to blend and verify that the chia seeds are not in any clusters.

Refrigerate the dish or jar for a minimum of 4 hours or overnight, covered. The liquid will be absorbed by the chia seeds during this time, giving them a pudding-like consistency.

If necessary, wash and cut the mixed berries. If you would like, you may gently crush some of the berries to release their juices.

Give the chia pudding a thorough stir when it has set. You may thin it out with a dash of milk if it's too thick.

Pour the pudding into jars or serving dishes.

Add as many more toppings as you want to the custard, such sliced almonds, shredded coconut or more mixed berries.

You can either serve the chia seed pudding with berries right away or keep it in the fridge for up to 4 days.
It's a tasty and healthy breakfast or snack option.
You can modify the sweetness or toppings to suit your tastes.

Greek Yoghurt Parfait with Granola

Ingredients:

- 1 cup of plain or flavoured Greek yoghurt, as desired
- Half a cup of granola, homemade or from the store
- Half a cup of mixed berries, including raspberries, blueberries and strawberries
- Maple syrup or honey *(optional; for drizzling)*
- Nuts or seeds *(for garnish, if desired)*

Instruction:

Start by adding a dollop of Greek yoghurt to the bottom of a serving glass or dish.

Sprinkle some oats over the yoghurt.

Spread some mixed berries over the granola.

Continue layering the ingredients until the glass or bowl is filled to your desired level or until you have used them all.

Drizzle some honey or maple syrup on top if you'd like it sweeter.

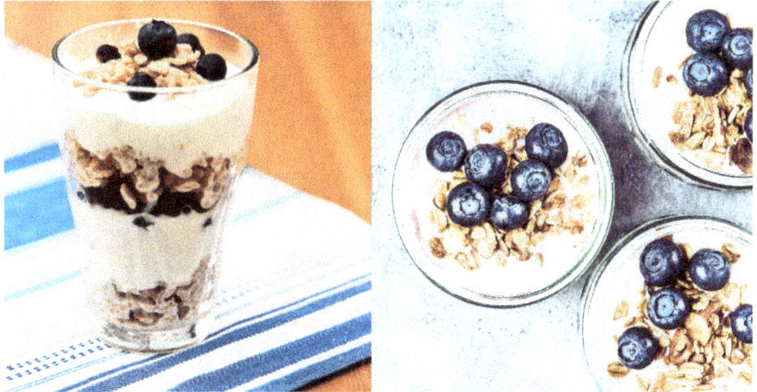

Add some nuts or seeds to the top for an added crunch and nutritional boost.

Serve this Greek Yoghurt Parfait with Granola right away.

You can easily alter this recipe by substituting other fruits, such chopped mangoes or sliced bananas and by experimenting with other yoghurt and granola flavours. It's an adaptable recipe that you may alter to fit your dietary requirements and taste preferences.

Banana Walnut Muffins

Ingredients:

- 1/2 cup of flour for all purposes
- One tsp baking powder
- One tsp baking soda
- Half a teaspoon of salt
- 3 mashed ripe bananas
- 3/4 cup of sugar, granulated
- 1/3 cup melted unsalted butter
- One big egg
- One tsp vanilla essence
- half a cup of walnuts, chopped

Instruction:

Set the oven temperature to 350°F (175°C).

Line a 12-cup muffin tray with paper liners or grease it.

Mix the flour, baking soda, baking powder and salt in a large basin.

The mashed bananas, sugar, melted butter, egg and vanilla extract should all be well mixed together in a separate basin.

Mix until well combined, pour the wet components into the dry ingredients. Take care not to overmix; a few lumps are OK.

Add the chopped walnuts and fold gently.

Using a spoon, pour the batter into each muffin tray, filling it approximately 3/4 of the way.

After 18 to 20 minutes of baking in a preheated oven, when 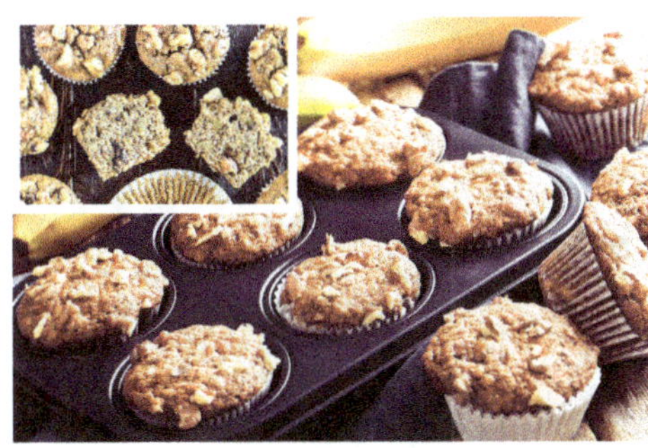 a toothpick is placed into the centre of a muffin, it should come out clean

After taking the muffins out of the oven, let them cool in the pan for a few minutes before moving them to a wire rack to finish cooling.

Let cool and then serve.

Spinach and Mushroom Frittata

Ingredients:

- 6 big eggs
- One cup of freshly chopped spinach
- One cup of sliced mushrooms
- ½ a cup of shredded cheese, either mozzarella or cheddar.
- 1/4 cup of cream or milk
- Two tsp olive oil
- One little onion, chopped
- 2 minced garlic cloves
- Salt and pepper.
- **Not required:** chopped fresh herbs for garnish, such as basil or parsley

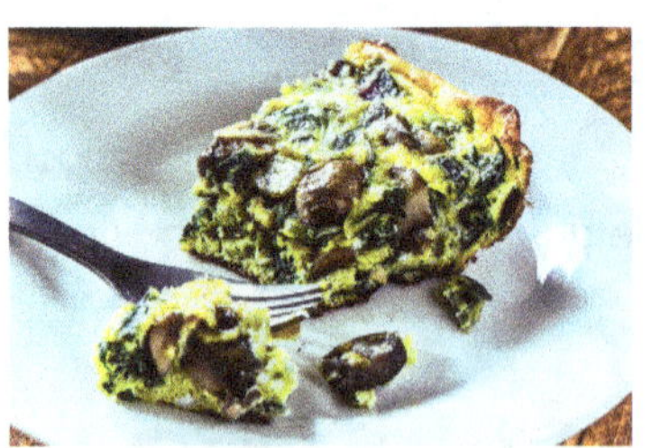

Instruction:

Turn the oven on to 375°F, or 190°C.

Whisk together the eggs and milk or cream in a large bowl. Add pepper and salt for seasoning.

In a skillet that is oven safe, warm the olive oil over medium heat. Add chopped onion and minced garlic and cook for 2 to 3 minutes or until softened and aromatic.

Sliced mushrooms should be added to the pan and cooked for 5 to 7 minutes or until they begin to exude moisture and soften.

Add the chopped spinach and simmer for approximately 2 minutes or until it wilts.

Evenly distribute the veggie mixture across the skillet. Over the veggies, pour the beaten eggs.

Let the mixture simmer for a few minutes, stirring occasionally, until the edges begin to solidify.

Evenly distribute shredded cheese on top of the frittata.

After transferring the pan to the oven, warm it and bake for 15 to 20 minutes or until the cheese is melted and bubbling and the eggs are set.

After the skillet is fully cooked, take it out of the oven and allow it to cool slightly before slicing it into wedges.

If preferred, garnish with finely chopped fresh herbs and serve warm. Savour your Frittata with spinach and mushrooms.

Overnight Oats with Almond Milk and Fruits

Ingredients:

- half a cup of rolled oats
- 1/2 cup almond milk *(amount to be adjusted according on personal liking)*
- One tablespoon of chia seeds *(optional; adds extra nutrients and texture)*
- One tablespoon honey or maple syrup, adjusted to taste
- One-fourth teaspoon of vanilla essence
- A little amount of salt
- your preferred choice of sliced fruits *(such as berries, bananas, apples, mangos, etc.)*
- Nuts or seeds *(optional)* as garnish

Instruction:

Place the rolled oats, almond milk, chia seeds *(if using)*, honey or maple syrup, vanilla essence and a little amount of salt in an airtight jar or mason jar. To equally mix all components, give it a good stir.

Top the oat mixture with your preferred cut fruits. Any fruit you choose or happen to have on hand may be used.

Sliced bananas, chopped apples or pieces of mango work nicely, as can berries like strawberries, blueberries or raspberries.

Stir the fruits gently into the oat mixture, then cover and refrigerate. Ensure that everything is well mixed.

Refrigerate the jar or container for at least 4–6 hours, preferably overnight, after sealing it. In this way, the oats may take in the liquid and become softer, till when you're ready to eat or the following morning.

The overnight oats may be eaten out of the jar or transferred to a bowl. For extra crunch and nutrients, you may optionally sprinkle some nuts or seeds on top.

You can alter your overnight oats to suit your own tastes. You may change the sweetness by adding different amounts of honey or maple syrup. Additionally, you may experiment with other nuts, seeds, fruits, and flavourings like cocoa powder or cinnamon.

Tofu Scramble with Peppers and Onions

Ingredients:

- One solid block of tofu
- One chopped bell pepper, any colour
- One chopped onion
- 2 minced garlic cloves
- Two tsp olive oil
- One tsp of turmeric
- Half a teaspoon of paprika
- Salt and pepper.
- **Optional:** chopped fresh herbs for garnish, such cilantro or parsley

Instruction:

Tofu should be pressed to eliminate extra moisture. To do this, cover the tofu block in paper towels or a fresh kitchen towel, then place something heavy on top.

Give it a good 15 to 20 minutes to sit.

Using your hands or a fork, crush the pounded tofu into little pieces.

In a big skillet over medium heat, warm up the olive oil. Add the chopped onions and bell peppers to the pan and cook for 5 to 7 minutes or until they are tender.

When aromatic, add the minced garlic to the pan and cook for an additional minute.

Stir the paprika and turmeric into the pan with the smashed tofu. In order to disperse the spices evenly, stir well to mix.

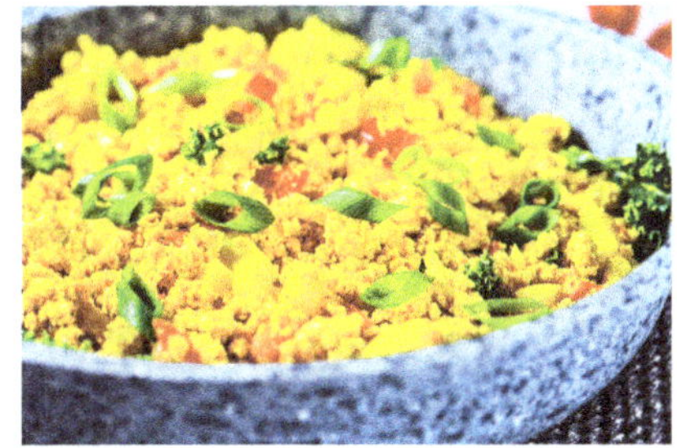

Cook - stirring occasionally until the tofu is cooked through and beginning to brown, approximately 5 to 7 minutes.

To taste, add salt and pepper for seasoning.

If desired, garnish with finely chopped fresh herbs.

Serve hot tofu scramble as a tasty and healthy choice for brunch or breakfast.

Vegan Breakfast Burrito

Ingredients:

- 1 cup of black beans, cooked
- 1 cup of potatoes, chopped
- 1 cup of chopped bell peppers, whichever colour you want
- one cup of finely chopped onions
- one cup of tomatoes, chopped
- 1 cup finely chopped kale or spinach
- 4 huge wheat tortillas
- One tablespoon of olive oil
- One teaspoon of cumin powder
- One tsp of paprika
- Salt and pepper.
- Avocado slices, salsa, spicy sauce and vegan cheese are *optional toppings*.

Instruction:

In a big skillet over medium heat, warm up the olive oil. Add the diced potatoes and simmer for approximately 5 minutes or until they begin to soften.

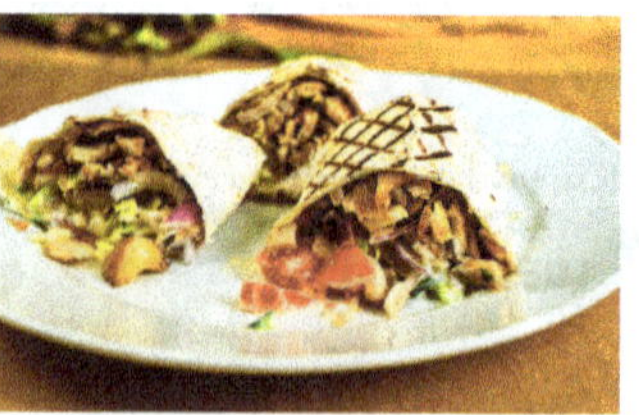

To the skillet, add the diced onions and bell peppers. Simmer for 5 to 7 minutes or until they are tender and have a hint of caramelization.

To the pan, add the diced tomatoes, ground cumin, paprika, black beans, salt and pepper. Make sure to thoroughly mix each component.

Cook for a further 2 to 3 minutes or until well heated.

Cook the chopped kale or spinach in the pan for one to two minutes or until it wilts and then take the skillet off of the hob.

To make the flour tortillas more malleable, reheat them in a different pan or the microwave for a brief period of time.

Place a spoonful of filling in the middle of each tortilla. Top with optional ingredients such vegan cheese, avocado slices, salsa or spicy sauce.

To construct a burrito, fold the tortilla's edges over the filling and roll it firmly.

Wrap each burrito in aluminium foil and keep it in the refrigerator for later use or serve right away.

Buckwheat Pancakes with Maple Syrup

Ingredients:

- One cup of buckwheat flour
- One tablespoon of optional sugar
- One tsp baking powder
- One-half tsp baking soda
- 1/4 tsp salt
- One cup of buttermilk *(or milk combined with one tablespoon of vinegar or lemon juice as an alternative)*
- One big egg
- Two teaspoons of oil or melted butter
- Maple syrup, suitable for serving

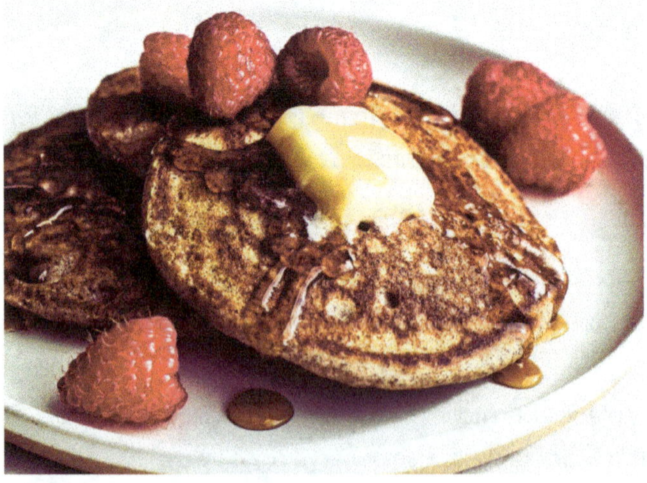

Instruction:

Mix the buckwheat flour, baking powder, baking soda, salt and sugar *(if using)* well in a large mixing dish.

Beat the egg, melted butter or oil and buttermilk together in a separate basin until smooth.

Mix until well combined then pour the wet components into the dry ingredients. *It's alright to have some lumps; don't overmix. Give the batter five to ten minutes to rest.*

Over medium heat, preheat a nonstick skillet or griddle. Grease lightly with oil or butter.

For each pancake, add about 1/4 cup of batter to the heated skillet. Simmer for 2 to 3 minutes or until surface bubbles appear and the edges seem firm.

After flipping, heat for a further 1 to 2 minutes - until the pancakes are cooked through and golden brown.

Grease the skillet as necessary and repeat with the remaining batter.

Drizzle the pancakes with maple syrup and serve warm.

Fruit Smoothie Bowl with Nut Butter

Ingredients:

Regarding the basis of the Smoothie:

- 1 frozen ripe banana
- One cup of mixed berries, including raspberries, blueberries and strawberries.
- half a cup of Greek yoghurt, plain
- 1/4 cup almond milk *(or any other kind of milk)*
- One tablespoon of **optionally** sweetened maple syrup or honey
- One tablespoon of nut butter *(almond or peanut butter, for example)*
- Half a teaspoon of **optional** vanilla essence

Regarding the Garnishes:

- Fresh fruits, cut into slices *(bananas, berries, kiwi, mango)*
- granola
- Chia seeds
- coconut shreds
- **Optional** nut butter drizzle
- **Optional:** honey or maple syrup for added sweetness

Instructions:

Blend together the frozen banana, mixed berries, Greek yoghurt, almond milk, nut butter, vanilla extract *(if desired)*, honey or maple syrup and almond milk in a blender.

Blend till creamy and smooth. ***If necessary,*** you may need to pause and scrape down the blender's sides.

Pour the smoothed-out smoothie base into a bowl.

Place your preferred toppings over the base of the smoothie. Use an assortment of fruits, nuts, seeds and granola; be creative with how they are arranged.

If desired, pour some more nut butter over top. For added sweetness, sprinkle some honey or maple syrup on top.

Enjoy this delectable Fruit Smoothie Bowl with Nut Butter right away.

You can alter this recipe to suit your dietary needs and taste preferences. Any mix of fruits and toppings is acceptable.

Zucchini and Carrot Fritters

Ingredients:

- One medium courgette
- one medium-sized carrot
- Half a cup of all-purpose flour
- 1/4 cup grated Parmesan cheese
- 2 chopped garlic cloves
- 2 beaten eggs
- Half a teaspoon of salt
- 1/4 tsp black pepper
- Olive oil for frying

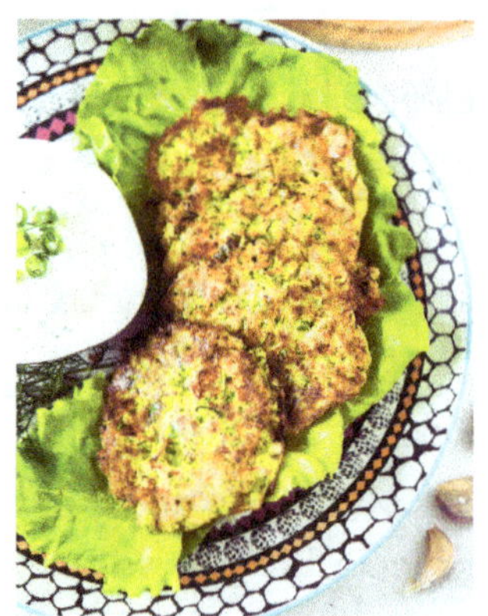

Instruction:

Utilising a food processor or a box grater, finely chop the carrot and zucchini. After grating the veggies, place them in a fresh cheesecloth or kitchen towel and press out as much liquid as you can.

Grated zucchini, carrot, flour, Parmesan cheese, minced garlic, beaten eggs, salt and black pepper should all be combined in a big mixing basin. Blend until well mix.

In a large skillet, heat a few tablespoons of olive oil over medium heat.

Using a spatula, gently flatten approximately 2 teaspoons of the fritter mixture into the pan. Ensure that there is enough room between each fritter.

Fry the fritters until they are crispy and golden brown, 3 to 4 minutes on each side. Depending on the size of your pan, you may have to fry them in batches.

After cooking, move the fritters to a platter covered with paper towels so that any extra oil may be drained off.

Enjoy the warm zucchini and carrot fritters on their own or with your preferred dipping sauce.

Breakfast Quiche with Sun-Dried Tomatoes

Ingredients:

- One pie crust, refrigerated *(homemade preferable)*
- 6 big eggs
- One cup of half-and-half
- One cup of shredded cheese, such Gruyere or cheddar

- ½ a cup Chopped sun-dried tomatoes *(drained if packaged in oil)*
- 1/4 cup of freshly chopped basil
- 1/4 cup of finely chopped green onions
- To taste, add salt and pepper.
- Cooked gammon or bacon, chopped mushrooms, spinach or any other preferred toppings ***are optional.***

Instruction:

Turn the oven on to 375°F or 190°C.

Press the pie dough into a 9-inch pie plate once it has been rolled out. Use a fork to prick the bottom, then bake for approximately 10 minutes or until the bottom is gently golden brown, then take out of the oven and set aside.

Beat the eggs well in a mixing dish. To taste, add salt and pepper for seasoning.

Evenly cover the bottom of the partly cooked pie crust with the shredded cheese.

Over the cheese layer, scatter the chopped sun-dried tomatoes, basil and green onions. Sprinkle any other ingredients, such as fried bacon or veggies, on top of the cheese.

Ensuring that the cheese and garnishes in the pie crust are properly distributed, carefully pour the egg mixture over them.

The quiche should be baked for 35 to 40 minutes or until the top is golden brown and the centre is set.

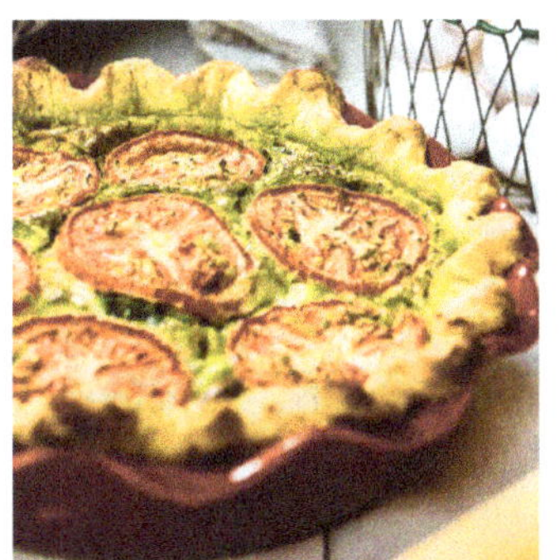

Before slicing and serving, take the cooked quiche out of the oven and allow it to cool for a few minutes.

Serve it warm, hot or even room temperature. It also makes excellent leftovers for simple, stress-free breakfasts all week long.

Veggie Breakfast Wrap with Hummus

Ingredients:

- One big tortilla made with spinach or whole wheat
- 2 to 3 tablespoons of hummus *(homemade or from the supermarket)*
- ¼ cup of bell peppers, chopped - any colour.

- ¼ cup of chopped tomatoes
- ¼ cup of cucumbers, chopped
- ¼ cup of carrots, shredded
- ¼ cup of chopped avocado
- handful of mixed greens or spinach
- Salt and pepper.
- Feta cheese, olives, sliced onions or any other vegetables of your choosing *are optional.*

Instruction:

To make the tortilla more malleable, warm it briefly in the microwave or on a pan.

Evenly cover the tortilla with hummus, leaving a half-inch border all around.

Arrange the shredded carrots, chopped bell peppers, tomatoes, cucumbers, avocado and mixed greens or spinach on top of the hummus.

To taste, add salt and pepper for seasoning.

Add whatever extras you'd like, like feta cheese, olives or sliced onions.

To wrap the contents, fold the tortilla's edges towards the centre and then firmly roll it up from the bottom.

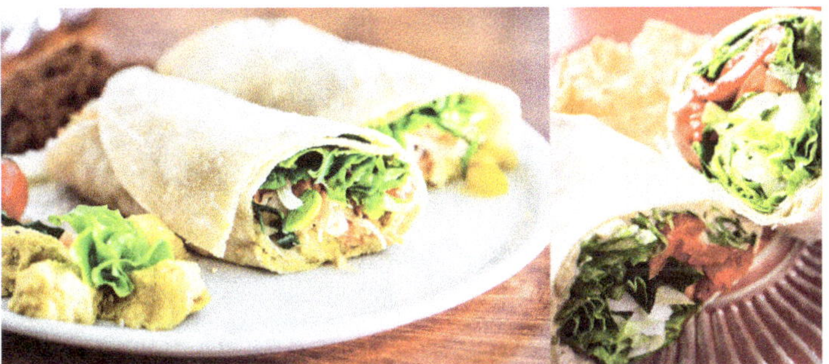

Cut the wrap in half diagonally, then serve right away.
Alternatively, wrap it in foil or parchment paper for an easy breakfast to-go.

Lentil Soup with Vegetables

Ingredients:

- One cup of washed and drained dry lentils
- One chopped onion
- 2 chopped carrots
- 2 chopped celery stalks
- 3 minced garlic cloves
- One can or fourteen ounces chopped tomatoes
- 6 cups vegetable broth
- 1 teaspoon each of ground coriander and cumin
- One-half tsp smoked paprika
- Salt and pepper.
- 2 tsp olive oil
- For garnish, use fresh cilantro or parsley **(optional)**.

Instruction:

In a big saucepan, warm the olive oil over medium heat. Add the celery, carrots and chopped onion.

Simmer for 5 to 7 minutes or until the veggies are tender, stirring periodically.

To the saucepan, add the minced garlic, smoked paprika, ground cumin and ground coriander. Cook until aromatic, one or two more minutes.

Pour the vegetable broth into the saucepan along with the washed lentils and chopped tomatoes *(with their juices)*. Mix well to blend.

After bringing the soup to a boil, lower the heat and simmer it for 25 to 30 minutes with a partly closed lid or until the lentils are soft.

Add salt and pepper to taste while preparing the soup. *As necessary,* adjust the seasoning.

You may puree some of the soup with an immersion blender to give it a little thicker consistency or you can leave it chunkier.

If preferred, top the hot lentil soup with chopped cilantro or fresh parsley and Serve.

The flavorful blend of veggies and spices in this lentil soup makes it filling and healthy. Feel free to alter the recipe to your liking by adding

Quinoa Salad with Roasted Vegetables

Ingredients:

- One cup of quinoa
- 2 cups of veggie broth or water
- 2 cups of diced, bite-sized mixed veggies *(such as red peppers, zucchini, cherry tomatoes, red onions, etc.)*
- Two tsp olive oil
- Salt and pepper.
- 1/4 cup finely chopped fresh herbs *(parsley, cilantro or basil)*
- One lemon's juice
- **Extra toppings:** avocado slices, feta cheese crumbles and roasted almonds or seeds

Instruction:

Set oven temperature to 400°F or 200°C.

To get rid of any bitterness, rinse the quinoa in a fine-mesh strainer with cold water.

Quinoa should be combined with water or vegetable broth in a saucepan. After bringing to a boil, lower the heat to a simmer, cover and cook the quinoa for about 15 minutes or until it is cooked through.

Take it off the heat and leave it covered for 5 minutes. Using a fork, fluff.

Toss chopped veggies with olive oil, salt and pepper on a baking sheet while the quinoa cooks. Make sure they are all in one layer.

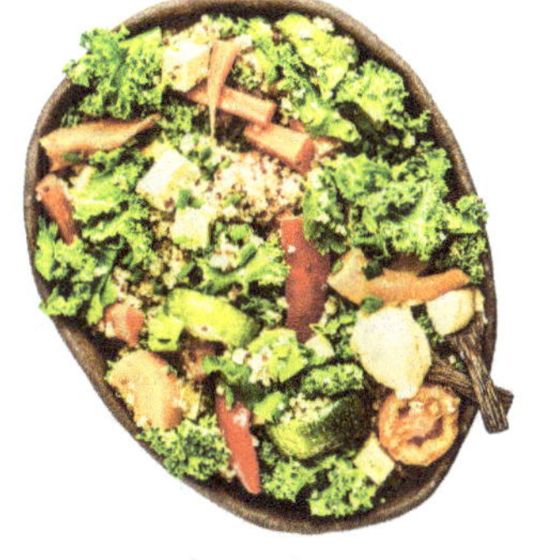

Bake the veggies for 20 to 25 minutes in a preheated oven, or until they are soft and have a hint of caramelization.

The cooked quinoa, chopped herbs, roasted veggies and lemon juice should all be combined in a big dish. Gently toss to mix. ***If necessary***, taste and adjust the seasoning.

Before serving, you may add sliced avocado, roasted nuts or seeds or crumbled feta cheese on top of the salad.

The quinoa salad may be served cold, room temperature or heated.

Chickpea Salad with Lemon-Tahini Dressing

Ingredients:

Regarding the Salad:

* 2 cans *(15 ounces each)* of chickpeas *(garbanzo beans)*
* 1 cucumber
* 1 diced bell pepper *(any colour)*
* 1 diced red onion
* 1 thinly sliced bell pepper
* 1 ¼ cup of freshly chopped parsley
* Salt and pepper.

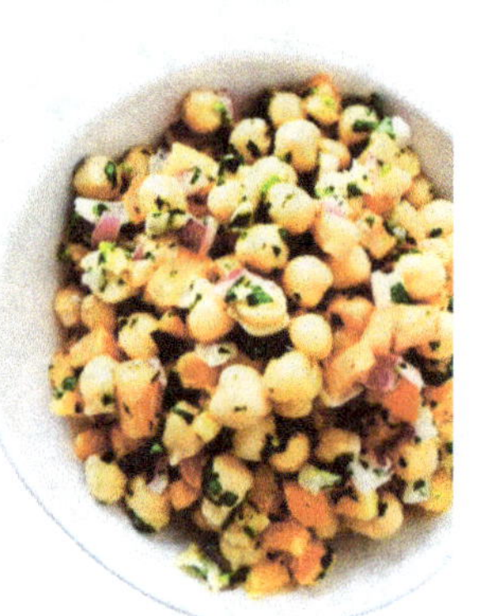

Regarding the Tahini-Lemon Dressing:

* One-fourth cup tahini
* 1/4 cup of freshly squeezed lemon juice
* Two tablespoons water
* One minced garlic clove
* One tablespoon of olive oil

- One tsp honey or maple syrup *(if desired)*
- Salt and pepper.

Instructions:

Drained and washed chickpeas.

Diced bell pepper, diced cucumber, sliced red onion and chopped fresh parsley should all be combined in a big dish.

Blend the tahini, water, fresh lemon juice, minced garlic, olive oil and honey or maple syrup *(if desired)* until a creamy consistency is achieved in a separate small bowl.

To taste, add salt and pepper for seasoning.

After adding the Lemon-Tahini Dressing to the chickpea salad, carefully spin everything to coat evenly.

If necessary, taste and adjust the seasoning by adding additional salt, pepper or lemon juice to suit your taste.

To enable the flavours to mingle, serve right away or chill for at least half an hour before serving. You may serve this salad cold or at room temperature.

Optional: Before serving, garnish with more finely chopped parsley or a sprinkling of sesame seeds.

Caprese Salad with Balsamic Glaze

Ingredients:

- One pound of fresh mozzarella cheese, cut
- 3 big ripe tomatoes, sliced
- fresh leaves of basil
- Salt and pepper.
- Extra virgin olive oil
- Balsamic reduction

Instruction:

Start by slicing the mozzarella cheese and tomatoes into uniform pieces that are about 1/4 inch thick.

On a serving dish, arrange the tomato and mozzarella slices alternately, slightly overlapping.

Place a few fresh basil leaves in between the mozzarella and tomato slices.

Over the salad, drizzle extra virgin olive oil. You may drizzle a lot of olive oil over the salad since it enhances its flavour.

To taste, add more salt and pepper to the salad.

Keep in mind that the cheese has a lot of salt already, so you may not need much.

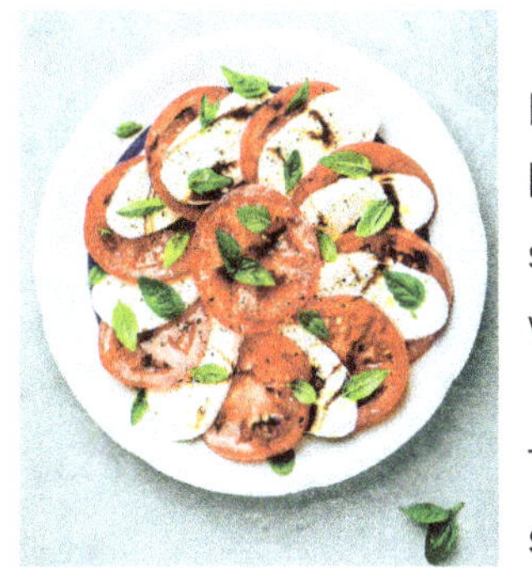

Finally, cover the salad with a balsamic glaze. To suit your taste, start with a smaller quantity and work your way up.

The balsamic glaze gives the salad a tart and sweet taste that goes well with its crisp texture.

Serve the caprese salad right away as a light snack or side dish.

Vegetable Stir-Fry with Tofu

Ingredients:

- One solid tofu block, drained and compressed
- Two tsp soy sauce

- One tablespoon of sesame oil
- One tablespoon of cornflour
- two tsp of vegetable oil
- Two cloves of garlic
- 1 minced one-inch piece of Ginger
- 1 minced onion
- 2 carrots chopped
- 1 bell pepper julienned
- one cup of broccoli florets
- One cup of trimmed snap peas
- 2 cups of cooked rice or noodles for serving

Regarding the Sauce:

- 3 tsp of soy sauce
- 2 tsp of hoisin sauce.
- One-tspn rice vinegar
- One-third cup brown sugar
- Two tablespoons of water
- 1 teaspoon of cornflour dissolved

Instruction:

To begin, prepare the tofu. Slice or cube the compressed tofu.

Combine 2 tablespoons soy sauce, 1 tablespoon sesame oil, and 1 tablespoon cornflour in a bowl.

Coat the tofu evenly by tossing it in this mixture. Give it a good 15 to 20 minutes to marinade.

Meanwhile, make the sauce by putting all of the ingredients in a small dish and setting them aside.

In a big skillet or wok, heat up one tablespoon of vegetable oil over medium-high heat.

Incorporate the marinated tofu and let it get crispy and golden brown on both sides. After taking the tofu out of the pan, set it aside.

If necessary, add one more tablespoon of vegetable oil to the same skillet. Add the ginger and garlic, minced and sauté until fragrant, approximately 1 minute.

To the skillet, add the bell pepper, broccoli florets, snap peas, sliced onion and julienned carrots.

Vegetables should be stir-fried for 3 to 4 minutes or until they begin to soften but maintain their crispness.

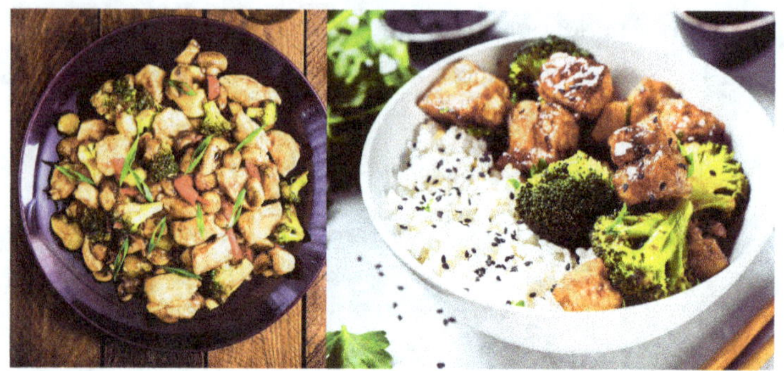

Place the cooked tofu back into the pan along with the veggies. After thoroughly mixing, pour the sauce over the tofu and veggies.

Simmer for a further 2 to 3 minutes or until the sauce has thickened and the food is well heated.

Serve hot tofu and vegetable stir-fry over prepared noodles or rice.

You are welcome to modify the veggies and sauce to suit your tastes.

Sweet Potato and Black Bean Quesadillas

Ingredients:

- Two medium-sized sweet potatoes, chopped and skinned
- One can (15 oz) of rinsed and drained black beans
- One cup of grated cheese *(mixture of Monterey Jack, cheddar, or blend)*
- 4 huge wheat tortillas
- 1 tsp of chilli powder
- ½ a teaspoon of cumin
- Salt and pepper.
- Cooking spray or olive oil

Extra toppings at your discretion:
→ Guacamole Salsa
→ sour cream
→ chopped cilantro
→ chopped tomatoes
→ Cut jalapeños

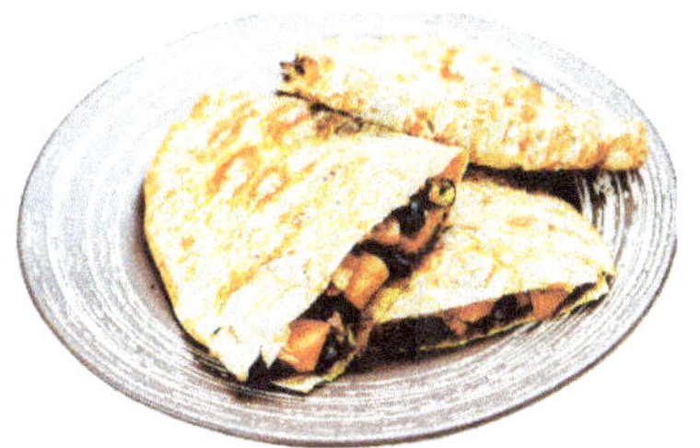

Instructions:

Set oven temperature to 400°F or 200°C.
Arrange the chopped sweet potatoes on a parchment paper-lined baking sheet.

Add a drizzle of olive oil, then season with salt, pepper, cumin and chilli powder then toss to coat.

Bake the sweet potatoes for 20 to 25 minutes or until they are soft and have a hint of caramelization, in the preheated oven.

Take them out of the oven and allow them to cool a little.

Using a fork or potato masher, mash the roasted sweet potatoes in a mixing basin.

After draining, add the black beans and stir until well mixed.

A big skillet should be heated to medium heat then spread a quarter of the sweet potato and black bean mixture equally over one side of a tortilla after placing it in the pan.

After spooning 1/4 of the shredded cheese over the sweet potato mixture, fold the remaining tortilla over the filling to form a half-moon.

Cook the quesadilla for 2 to 3 minutes on each side or until the cheese has melted and the tortilla is crispy and golden brown.

Continue this process with the remaining tortillas and filling.

After they are done, move the quesadillas to a chopping board and cut them into wedges.

Serve the quesadillas warm, garnished with your preferred salsa, guacamole, sour cream, diced tomatoes, chopped cilantro or sliced jalapeños.

Greek Salad with Tzatziki Dressing

Ingredients for Salad dressing:

- Two big tomatoes
- diced red onion
- diced cucumber
- diced green bell pepper - finely sliced
- diced 1/2 cup Kalamata olives
- 200g of pitted feta cheese
- 1/4 cup chopped fresh parsley and crumbled
- Salt and pepper.
- **Optional:** For extra protein, try one cup of cooked chickpeas or grilled chicken.

Ingredients for the Dressing Tzatziki:

- One cup of Greek yoghurt
- half of a cucumber, drained and shredded

- 2 minced garlic cloves
- One tablespoon of freshly squeezed lemon juice
- One tablespoon of extra virgin olive oil
- One tablespoon of freshly chopped dill
- Salt and pepper.

Instructions:

Diced tomatoes, cucumber, red onion, bell pepper, Kalamata olives and *optional* grilled chicken or chickpeas should all be combined in a big salad dish.

To create the tzatziki dressing, combine the Greek yoghurt, chopped dill, olive oil, minced garlic and shredded cucumber in a separate bowl.

To taste, add salt and pepper for seasoning.

Drizzle the salad items with the tzatziki dressing and gently mix to coat.

Top the salad with the chopped parsley and crumbled feta cheese.

If necessary, add more salt and pepper for seasoning.
To let the flavours melt together, serve right away or let it sit in the fridge for half an hour before serving.

Ingredients:

- Four big bell peppers of any hue
- Two tsp olive oil
- One little onion, cut finely
- two minced garlic cloves
- Four cups freshly chopped, roughly-cut spinach leaves
- One cup of cooked rice or quinoa
- One cup of feta cheese, crumbled
- 1/4 cup of Parmesan cheese, grated
- Salt and pepper.
- One tsp of dehydrated Oregano
- half a teaspoon of dried basil
- 1/4 tsp *optional* red pepper flakes
- 1/4 cup of freshly chopped parsley, for decoration

Instruction:

Turn the oven on to 375°F, or 190°C.

Slice off the bell peppers' tops, then take out the seeds and membranes. After rinsing them with cold water, put them aside.

In a big skillet over medium heat, warm up the olive oil.

Add the chopped onion and garlic and cook for 3–4 minutes or until softened.

Cook the chopped spinach in the pan for 2 to 3 minutes or until it wilts.

Cooked quinoa or rice, sautéed spinach combination, grated Parmesan cheese, crumbled feta cheese, dried oregano, dried basil and red pepper flakes *(if used)* should all be combined in a big mixing basin.

Toss to blend thoroughly.

Gently push down to cram the spinach and feta mixture into each bell pepper.

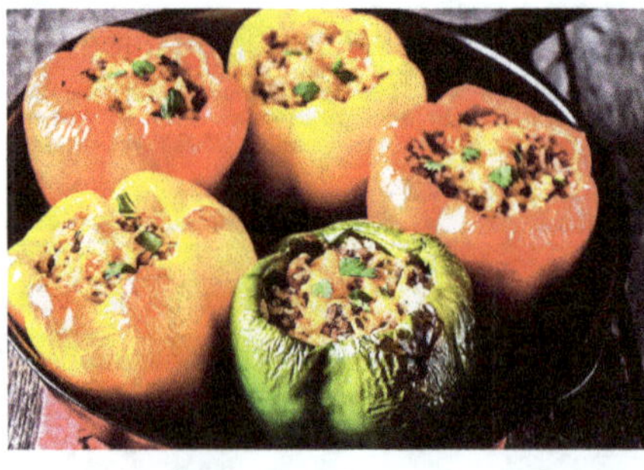

The filled peppers should be put on a roasting tray.

To make each pepper stand straight in the plate, you may cut a little bit off the bottom if needed.

Bake the baking dish in the preheated oven for 25 to 30 minutes or until the peppers are soft, covered with aluminium foil.

After taking off the foil, bake the peppers for a further 5 to 10 minutes or until the tops begin to turn a light golden brown.

When finished, take it out of the oven and let it cool down for a few minutes.

Before serving, sprinkle some freshly chopped parsley on top.

Mushroom Barley Risotto

Ingredients:

- One cup of pearl barley
- 4 cups of veggie broth
- 2 teaspoons of olive oil
- One onion, chopped finely
- 8 ounces of sliced mushrooms *(like cremini or shiitake)*
- 2 chopped garlic cloves
- Half a cup of dry white wine, ***if desired***
- 1/4 cup of ***optionally*** grated Parmesan cheese
- Salt and pepper.

- Chopped fresh parsley *(for garnish)*

Instruction:

Simmer the vegetable broth over medium heat in a medium saucepan. While you make the risotto, keep it warm.

Heat the olive oil in a large separate skillet over medium heat. Add the chopped onion and garlic and cook for 3–4 minutes or until they are transparent.

After adding the sliced mushrooms to the pan, heat for 5 to 6 minutes or until they are soft and browned.

Add the pearl barley and simmer, stirring frequently, for a further 2 to 3 minutes or until the barley is gently toasted.

Add the white wine, *if using,* and heat, stirring from time to time, until the liquid is largely absorbed.

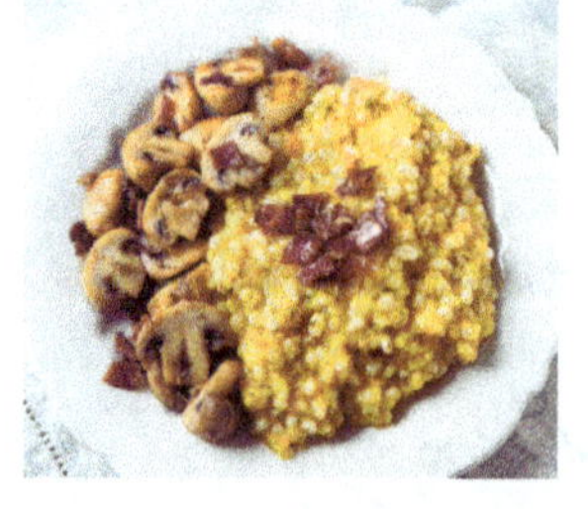

One ladleful at a time, add the heated vegetable broth to the pan, stirring constantly and letting each addition soak before adding more.

This procedure should be repeated until the barley is creamy and soft, around 30 to 40 minutes.

Grated Parmesan cheese, *if needed,* should be added after the barley has reached the required consistency.

To taste, add salt and pepper for seasoning.

Garnish the heated mushroom barley risotto with freshly chopped parsley.

Eggplant Parmesan with Marinara Sauce

Ingredients:

Regarding the Marinara Sauce:

- 2 tsp olive oil
- 4 minced garlic cloves
- 1 little onion, diced finely
- 1 can (28 oz) of chopped tomatoes
- 1 tsp of dehydrated oregano
- 1 tsp of dried basil
- Salt and pepper.
- A pinch of sugar, *if desired*

- Two medium eggplants cut into rounds of half an inch
- Salt
- 2 cups of breadcrumbs
- Grated Parmesan cheese, 1 cup
- 2 big, beaten eggs
- One cup of flour for all purposes
- Olive oil for frying
- 2 cups of mozzarella cheese, shredded
- **As a garnish,** fresh basil leaves

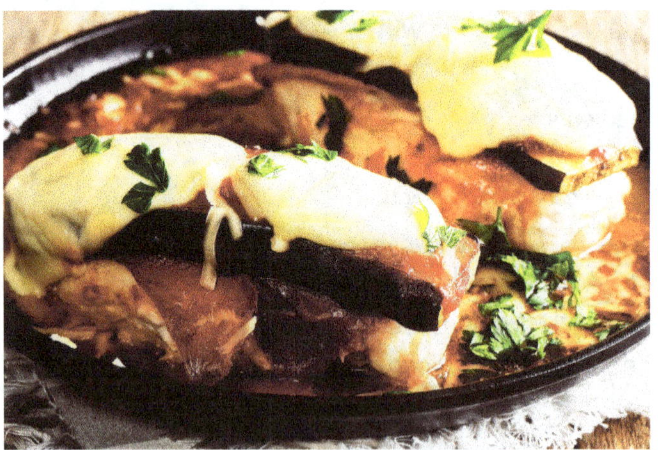

Instructions:

For the Marinara Sauce:

In a big saucepan set over medium heat, warm the olive oil.

Add chopped onion and minced garlic and sauté for approximately 5 minutes or until the onion is tender and aromatic.

Add the smashed tomatoes, sugar *(if using)*, salt, pepper, dried oregano and dried basil.

Once the sauce reaches a simmer, cook it for 15 to 20 minutes, stirring now and again.

Taste and adjust the seasoning.

Regarding the Parmesan aubergine:

Turn the oven on to 375°F, or 190°C.

Arrange the cut eggplants onto a baking sheet and lightly dust both surfaces with sea salt.

To extract moisture, let them sit for around thirty minutes. Using paper towels, pat the eggplant slices dry to absorb any remaining moisture.

Arrange the flour, beaten eggs and breadcrumbs with grated Parmesan cheese in three different shallow bowls.

Each aubergine slice should be floured, dipped in beaten eggs and then covered with breadcrumb mixture.

In a big skillet set over medium-high heat, warm up the olive oil. Slices of breaded aubergine should be fried in batches for 2 to 3 minutes on each side or until golden brown.

To drain excess oil, transfer to a plate lined with paper towels.

Line the bottom of a baking dish with a thin layer of marinara sauce. Put a few slices of cooked aubergine on top.

Drizzle the eggplant slices with more marinara sauce and top with mozzarella cheese shreds.

Continue layering until all of the eggplant pieces have been utilised. Top with a layer of mozzarella cheese and marinara sauce.

Bake the baking dish in the preheated oven for about 25 to 30 minutes or until the cheese is bubbling and melted, covered with aluminium foil.

After 5 to 10 more minutes, remove the foil and continue baking the cheese until it becomes golden brown.

Before serving, garnish with fresh basil leaves.

Cauliflower Fried Rice

Ingredients:

- One medium cauliflower head
- Two tsp of sesame oil
- two minced garlic cloves
- One little onion, chopped
- One cup of mixed veggies, including sliced bell peppers, peas, carrots and corn
- 2 gently beaten eggs
- 3 tsp of soy sauce
- Salt and pepper.
- **Garnishes optional:** Chopped cilantro, sesame seeds and sliced green onions

Instruction:

After chopping the cauliflower into florets, pulse it in a food processor until the pieces resemble rice. *Take care not to overprocess it to the point of mushiness.*

In a large pan or wok, heat 1 tablespoon of sesame oil over medium-high heat.

Add the chopped onion and minced garlic and sauté for two to three minutes or until the onion becomes translucent.

When the mixed veggies are soft, add them to the pan and simmer for 3–4 minutes.

Transfer the veggies to one side of the pan and cover the empty side with the beaten eggs. Let them simmer, stirring now and again, until well cooked and scrambled.

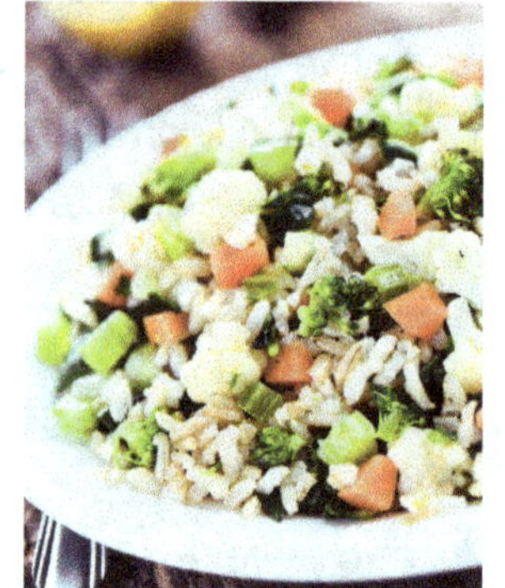

Mix the veggies in the pan with the scrambled eggs.

Add the remaining tablespoon of sesame oil, soy sauce and cauliflower "rice" to the pan. Toss to thoroughly mix in all the ingredients.

Cook for approximately 5 to 7 minutes, stirring regularly or until the cauliflower is soft but still somewhat crunchy.

To taste, add salt and pepper for seasoning.

If preferred, garnish with chopped cilantro, sesame seeds and green onion slices and serve.

Falafel Wraps with Hummus and Veggies

Ingredients:

- 1 cup of overnight-soaked dry chickpeas
- One little onion, finely sliced
- 2 minced garlic cloves
- 1/4 cup finely chopped fresh parsley
- One teaspoon of cumin powder
- One tsp finely ground coriander
- One-half tsp baking powder
- Salt and pepper.
- For frying, use olive oil
- Regular or whole wheat wraps
- Hummus *(homemade or from the shop)*
- Cucumber slices
- Slices of Tomatoes
- Shredded green leafy vegetables
- Pickled turnips, tahini sauce and spicy sauce are **optional.**

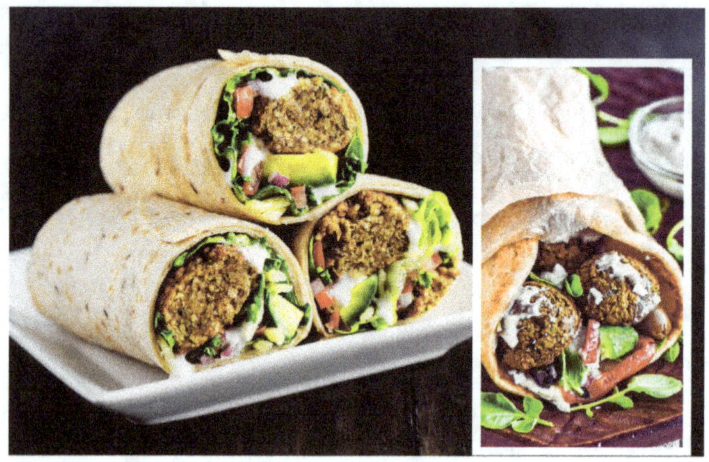

Instruction:

After soaking, drain and rinse the chickpeas.

The chickpeas, onion, garlic, parsley, cumin, coriander, baking powder, salt and pepper should all be combined in a food processor. Pulse the mixture until it's thoroughly blended but still gritty.

It may be necessary for you to scrape down the food processor bowl's sides many times.

The falafel mixture should be poured into a bowl and chilled for at least half an hour. This will facilitate the mixture's firming up and shaping.

Meanwhile, wash and slice the veggies in preparation for the falafel mixture. Also, *if preferred,* reheat the wraps in a pan or microwave.

In a pan over medium heat, warm the olive oil. Form the cold falafel mixture into a small patty using approximately 2 teaspoons.

The falafel patties should be fried for 3 to 4 minutes on each side or until they are crispy and golden brown on both sides. *The size of your pan may determine whether you need to cook them in batches.*

After cooking, take the falafel patties out of the pan and drain them on paper towels to get rid of any leftover oil.

Drizzle each wrap with a good dollop of hummus to assemble.

Top with a few falafel patties, sliced cucumbers, tomatoes, shredded lettuce and any other toppings *(pickled turnips, tahini sauce, spicy sauce, etc.)* that you'd like.

Serve the wraps right away after carefully rolling them up and tucking in the sides.

Tomato Basil Bruschetta

Ingredients:

- 4-5 chopped ripe tomatoes
- 1/4 cup finely chopped fresh basil leaves
- 2 minced garlic cloves
- 2 teaspoons pure olive oil
- One-third cup balsamic vinegar
- Salt and pepper.
- One baguette, cut into slices
- Using olive oil to brush

Instruction:

Turn the oven on to 375°F, or 190°C.

Diced tomatoes, minced garlic, chopped basil, extra virgin olive oil, balsamic vinegar, salt and pepper should all be combined in a mixing dish.

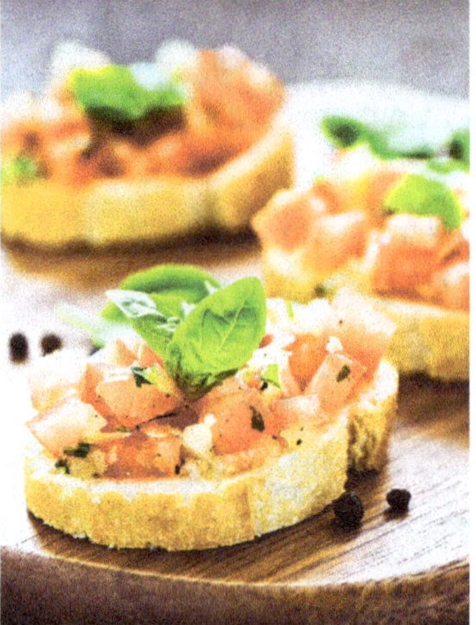

Toss to blend thoroughly.

As you make the bread, let the tomato mixture marinade.

Cut the baguette into slices that are 1/2 inch thick. Arrange the slices in a single layer on a baking sheet.

Apply a thin layer of olive oil on both sides of every bread piece.

After preheating the oven, place the baking sheet inside and bake for 5 to 7 minutes or until the bread is just beginning to brown.

After taking the toast out of the oven, allow it to cool for a little while.

After the sauce has cooled down a little, liberally pour it over each piece of bread.

Serve this mouthwatering Tomato Basil Bruschetta right away.

You can modify the seasoning to suit your tastes. If you'd like, you may also top it with a little grated Parmesan cheese for more flavour.

Quinoa and Black Bean Stuffed Peppers

Ingredients:

- 4 big bell peppers, diced to your desired colour
- 1 cup of washed Quinoa
- One can *(15 ounces)* of rinsed and drained black beans
- One cup of fresh, frozen or canned Corn kernels
- One little onion, chopped
- two minced garlic cloves
- One teaspoon of cumin powder
- One tsp of chilli powder
- To taste, add salt and pepper.
- One cup of shredded cheese (you may use Monterey Jack, cheddar, or another favourite)
- **Extra toppings at your discretion:** sliced avocado, chopped cilantro, salsa and sour cream

Instruction:

Turn the oven on to 375°F or 190°C. Grease a baking dish that can accommodate the peppers.

Remove the bell peppers' seeds and membranes by cutting off the tops. *If required,* thinly slice the bottoms of the peppers to enable them to sit erect in the baking dish.

After preparing the baking dish, place the peppers in it and set aside.

Add the two cups of water and the quinoa to a medium-sized pot. After bringing to a boil, lower the heat to a simmer, cover and cook the quinoa for about 15 minutes or until it is tender and the water has been absorbed.

Take off the stove and use a fork to fluff the quinoa.

Heat some olive oil in a big skillet over medium heat.

Cook chopped onion for about 5 minutes or until it is tender.

Add the chilli powder, powdered cumin and minced garlic; simmer for an additional minute or until fragrant.

To the pan with the onions and spices, add the cooked quinoa, black beans and corn. Cook for a few more minutes until well cooked, stirring carefully to incorporate.

To taste, add salt and pepper for seasoning.

Fill the prepped bell peppers with the quinoa and black bean mixture, gently pushing down to compact the filling.

Top each filled pepper with grated cheese.

When the oven is ready, bake the baking dish covered with aluminium foil for 25 to 30 minutes or until the cheese is melted and bubbling and the peppers are soft.

If preferred, remove the foil and bake for a further 5 minutes to gently brown the cheese.

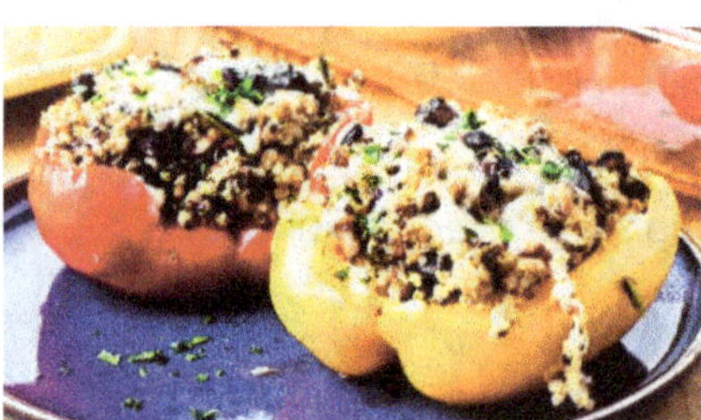

Serve the filled peppers hot with optional toppings like sliced avocado, salsa, sour cream or chopped cilantro.

Veggie Sushi Rolls with Soy Sauce

Ingredients:

Regarding the Sushi rice:

- 2 cups of sushi rice
- 2 and a half cups water
- one-third cup rice vinegar
- 2 tsp sugar

- One tsp salt

Regarding the Sushi rolls:

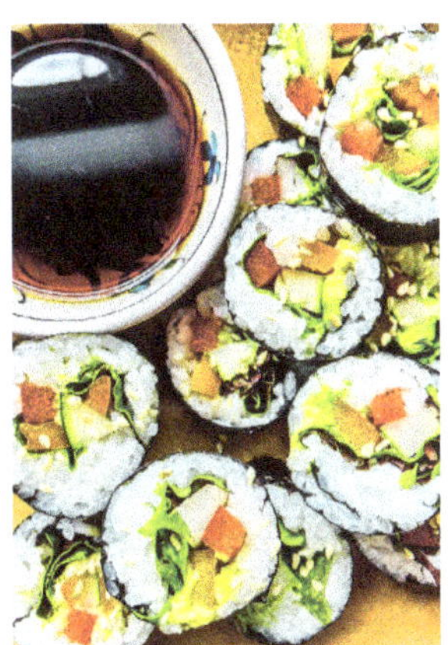

- Sheets of nori seaweed
- a variety of veggies *(include tofu, cucumber, avocado, carrot and/or bell pepper)*
- Sushi rolling mat made of bamboo
- **For serving,** Soy sauce
- **For serving,** pickled ginger and wasabi are *optional.*

Instruction:

Till the water runs clear - rinse the sushi rice under cold water.

In a rice cooker or saucepan, combine the rinsed rice with water and cook as directed on the box.

Make the sushi vinegar combination while the rice is cooking. Combine the sugar, salt and rice vinegar in a small pot.

Cook over low heat until the salt and sugar are completely dissolved. Take off the heat and let it cool.

After the rice has cooked, pour it into a big basin and whisk in the sushi vinegar mixture very carefully.

Take care not to crush the grains of rice. Let the rice cool until it reaches room temperature.

Cut the veggies into thin strips and set aside while the rice cools.

Arrange a nori sheet on the bamboo sushi rolling mat, shiny side down. To ensure that the sushi rice does not adhere to the nori, wet your hands with water and uniformly distribute a thin coating of rice, leaving a 1-inch border at the top edge.

Lay down the veggies you want in a line in the middle of the rice.

Roll the sushi firmly from the bottom edge, tucking in the contents with your fingers as you roll, using the bamboo mat as a guide.

After the roll has been rolled, compress and shape it using the bamboo mat.

Cut the sushi roll into bite-sized pieces using a sharp knife.
To keep the knife from sticking, dip it into water in between
each slice.

Serve the vegetable sushi rolls with a side of pickled ginger
and wasabi and soy sauce for dipping.

Butternut Squash Soup with Croutons

Ingredients:

Regarding the Soup:

- One medium-sized butternut squash that has been peeled, seeded and diced.
- One chopped onion
- 2 minced garlic cloves
- 4 cups of chicken or veggie stock
- 1 tsp finely ground cinnamon
- 1 ½ tsp ground nutmeg
- Salt and pepper.
- Two tsp olive oil

Regarding the Croutons:

- 2 cups of cubed bread *(better if the bread is a day old)*
- 2 tsp olive oil
- half a teaspoon of powdered garlic
- Salt and pepper.

Instruction:

Turn the oven on to 375°F, or 190°C.

Heat two tablespoons of olive oil in a big saucepan over medium heat.

Add the minced garlic and onion, sauté for approximately five minutes or until the ingredients are tender.

Add the cubed butternut squash, salt, pepper, ground nutmeg and cinnamon to the saucepan. Mix everything together.

Add the chicken or vegetable broth and heat the mixture until it boils. After the squash reaches a boil, lower the heat to a simmer, cover and let it cook for 20 to 25 minutes or until it becomes soft.

Make the croutons while the soup is boiling. Toss the cubed bread with 2 tablespoons olive oil, salt, pepper and garlic powder in a mixing bowl until well covered.

Arrange the bread cubes that have been seasoned in a single layer on a baking pan. The croutons should bake for 10 to 15 minutes in a preheated oven or until they are crispy and golden brown.

After the butternut squash is soft, puree the soup until it's smooth using an immersion blender.

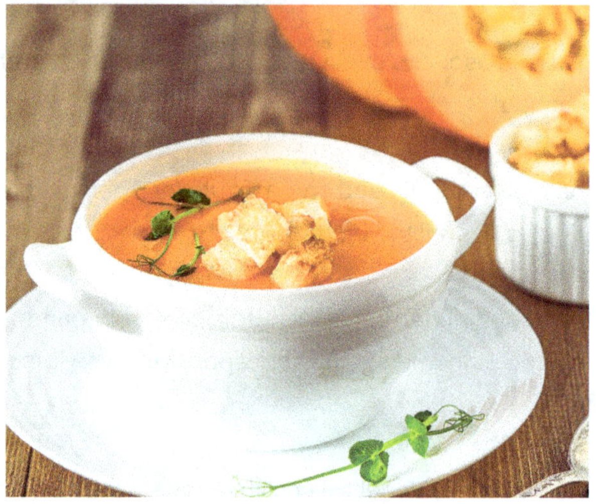

As an alternative, you may transfer the soup to a blender in stages and process it until it's smooth.

If needed, taste the soup and adjust the seasoning.

Serve the hot butternut squash soup with the cooked croutons on top as a garnish.

To suit your tastes, feel free to change the seasonings or add more herbs or spices.

Ratatouille with Herbed Couscous

Ingredients:

Regarding Ratatouille:

- One eggplant
- Two diced zucchinis
- One chopped onion
- 2 diced red peppers *(orange, yellow or red)*
- 3 diced garlic cloves
- 3 minced tomatoes
- 2 diced tablespoons tomato paste
- Two tsp olive oil
- A single tsp of dried thyme
- One tsp of dehydrated oregano
- Salt and pepper.

For the Couscous with herbs:

- One cup of couscous
- 1/4 cup water or vegetable broth
- Two tsp olive oil
- One tablespoon of freshly chopped Parsley
- One tablespoon of freshly chopped Basil
- Salt and pepper.

Instructions:

In a big skillet, warm the olive oil over medium heat.

Saute the minced garlic and chopped onion for two to three minutes or until the ingredients become tender.

To the pan, add the diced zucchini, bell peppers, eggplant, oregano, thyme and salt and pepper. Simmer for 10 to 12 minutes or until the veggies are soft, stirring once and again.

Add the tomato paste and diced tomatoes and stir. Allow the flavours to mingle by cooking for a further five minutes.

Taste and adjust seasoning.

In the meanwhile, get the herbed couscous ready. Bring the water or vegetable broth to a boil in a saucepan.

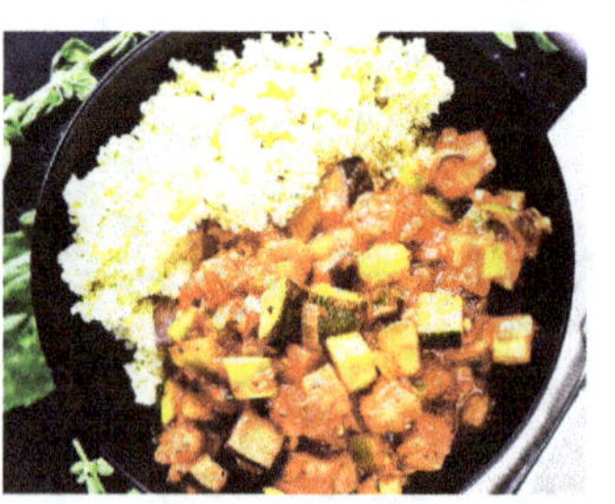

Remove from heat, cover and stir in the couscous. Allow to sit until the liquid is absorbed, approximately 5 minutes.

Using a fork, fluff the couscous and mix in the olive oil, salt, pepper, chopped parsley and chopped basil.

Over the herbed couscous, serve the ratatouille. *If preferred,* you may add more fresh herbs as a garnish.

Vegetable Lasagna with Cashew Cheese

Ingredients:

Regarding the Cashew Cheese:

- One cup of uncooked cashews that have been soaked in water for 4 or more hours
- 1/4 cup of nutritional yeast
- 2 tsp lemon juice
- 1 minced garlic clove
- Salt and pepper.
- Water, as required to change the consistency

For the Lasagna with Vegetables:

- One box (12–16 oz) lasagna noodles *(if necessary, substitute gluten-free noodles)*
- Two tsp olive oil
- One chopped onion
- 3 Garlic cloves
- 2 Zucchinis chopped
- 1 Bell pepper chopped

- 1 cup mushrooms diced
- Two cups Spinach leaves sliced
- Two cups of Marinara sauce
- Salt and pepper.
- Chop some fresh Basil leaves *(optional for garnish)*

Instructions:

Turn the oven on to 375°F or 190°C.

As directed on the box, cook the lasagna noodles until they are al dente. After draining - set aside.

The soaked cashews, nutritional yeast, lemon juice, minced garlic, salt, pepper and a little amount of water should all be combined in a food processor or blender.

In order to get a creamy consistency, add more water as necessary and blend until smooth. Put aside.

Heat the olive oil in a big skillet over medium heat. Add chopped onion and minced garlic and cook for 3–4 minutes or until softened and aromatic.

To the pan, add the sliced mushrooms, bell pepper and chopped zucchini. Cook the veggies for a further 5 to 6 minutes or until they are soft.

Cook the spinach leaves in the pan for approximately 2 minutes or until they have wilted. To taste, add salt and pepper for seasoning.

Line a 9 x 13-inch baking dish with a thin coating of marinara sauce.

Cover the marinara sauce with a layer of cooked lasagna noodles.

Cover the noodles with a coating of cashew cheese and then a layer of the cooked veggie mixture.

Once all the ingredients have been used, repeat the layers: marinara sauce, noodles, cashew cheese and veggies. End with a layer of marinara sauce on top.

Bake the lasagna in the preheated oven for thirty to thirty-five minutes, or until it's hot and bubbling. Cover the baking dish with foil.

Take off the foil and bake for a further 5 to 10 minutes or until a light golden colour appears on top.

When finished, take it out of the oven and allow it to cool down before slicing.

If preferred, garnish with finely chopped fresh basil leaves just before serving.

Stuffed Portobello Mushrooms with Quinoa and Spinach

Ingredients:

- 4 substantial Portobello mushrooms
- 1 cup of quinoa
- 2 cups water or vegetable broth
- 2 cups finely chopped fresh spinach
- One little onion, diced finely
- 2 minced garlic cloves
- One tablespoon of Olive oil
- Grated Parmesan cheese, 1/2 cup *(optional)*
- Salt and pepper.
- Garnish with fresh Parsley or Basil *(optional)*.

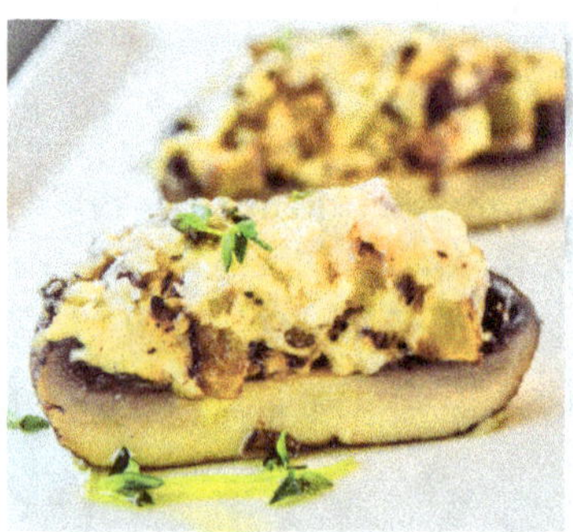
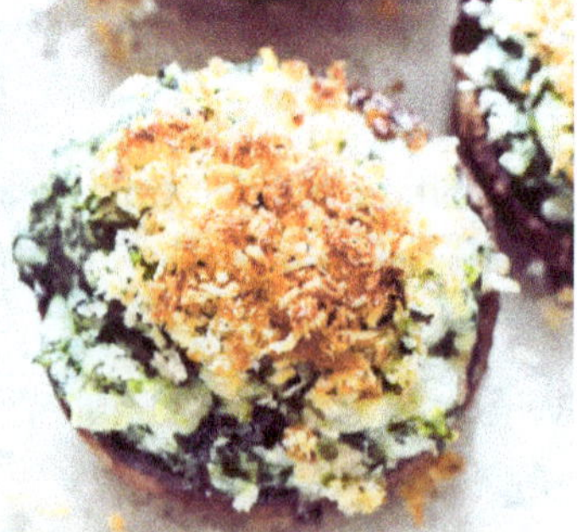

Instruction:

Turn the oven on to 375°F, or 190°C.

In order to get rid of any bitterness, rinse the quinoa in cold water.

Heat the vegetable broth *(or water)* in a medium-sized pot until it boils.

After adding the quinoa, lower the heat to low, cover and simmer the quinoa for 15 to 20 minutes or until it is cooked through and all of the liquid has been absorbed.

Take off the heat and use a fork to fluff.

Remove the stems from the Portobello mushrooms and use a spoon to carefully scrape out the gills while the quinoa cooks.

Arrange the mushrooms on a baking sheet that has been gently oiled or covered with parchment paper.

Heat the olive oil in a pan over medium heat. Add the chopped onion and garlic and cook for 3–4 minutes or until softened.

Cook the chopped spinach in the pan for 2 to 3 minutes or until it wilts.

Put the cooked quinoa and spinach mixture into a big bowl. To taste, add salt and pepper for seasoning.

Fill each Portobello mushroom cap with a spoonful of the quinoa and spinach mixture, gently pushing down to compact the filling.

Garnish each filled mushroom with grated Parmesan cheese, *if desired.*

Bake for 20 to 25 minutes or until the mixture is cooked through and the mushrooms are soft.

Take out of the oven and if you'd like, top with some fresh basil or parsley before serving.

Thai Green Curry with Tofu and Vegetables

Ingredients:

Regarding the Curry paste:

- 2–3 chopped green Thai chilies *(adjust to taste)*

- Two sliced lemongrass stalks *(only the white portion)*
- 4 minced garlic cloves
- 1 chopped shallot
- 1 chopped ginger piece the size of a thumb
- One bunch of fresh Cilantro with distinct branches and leaves
- 2 teaspoons of freshly chopped Basil leaves
- One tablespoon of finely chopped, fresh mint leaves
- One teaspoon each of Ground Cumin and Coriander
- One tsp powdered turmeric
- 1 lime's juice and zest
- Two tsp soy sauce
- 1 ⅓ cup brown sugar
- Salt to taste.

Regarding the Curry:

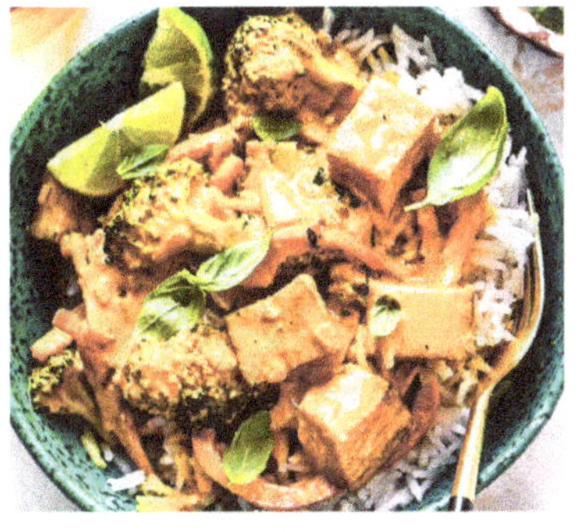

- One block of diced and pressed firm Tofu
- 2 cups chopped mixed veggies *(broccoli, carrots, bell peppers, snow peas and zucchini)*
- One can (14 oz) milk from Coconuts
- One cup of broth made with vegetables
- 2 teaspoons of frying oil
- Hot jasmine rice, ready to be served

Instructions:

To make the curry paste, put all the ingredients in a food
processor or blender and pulse until smooth.

To make sure everything is well combined, you may need to
scrape down the bowl's sides a few times.

In a large skillet or wok, heat the oil over medium heat.

After adding the tofu cubes, heat for 5 to 7 minutes or until
golden brown on both sides. Take out the tofu and put it
aside in a skillet.

If necessary, add a bit of extra oil to the same pan and add the
curry paste. Cook, stirring regularly for 2 to 3 minutes or until
aromatic.

When the mixed veggies are added to the pan, toss them to
evenly cover them with curry paste.

Add the veggie broth and coconut milk. Once the mixture
reaches a simmer, cook it for 5 to 7 minutes or until the
veggies are soft.

Return the cooked tofu to the skillet and mix everything together. To thoroughly heat the tofu, cook for a further 2 to 3 minutes.

If necessary, taste and adjust the flavour with more soy sauce or salt.

Serve hot over cooked jasmine rice, **If preferred,** top hot dish with lime wedges and fresh cilantro leaves.

Eggplant and Chickpea Tagine

Ingredients:

- One big eggplant, chopped
- One can (15 oz.) of washed and drained chickpeas
- One sliced onion
- 2 minced garlic cloves
- One can (14.5 oz) chopped tomatoes
- One teaspoon of cumin powder
- One tsp finely ground coriander
- half a teaspoon of cinnamon powder
- ¼ tsp ground ginger
- ¼ teaspoon cayenne *(optional; add more spice if desired)*
- Salt and pepper.
- 2 tsp olive oil

- ¼ cup of finely chopped fresh parsley or cilantro, for garnish
- Cooked rice or Couscous for serving.

Instruction:

In a big skillet or tagine, warm up the olive oil over medium heat.

Add minced garlic and sliced onion to the skillet. Sauté for 3–4 minutes or until the onion is transparent.

Cook the chopped aubergine in the pan for 5 to 7 minutes or until it begins to soften.

Add the ground ginger, cinnamon, cumin and coriander, as well as the cayenne pepper *(if using)*. Simmer for a further one to two minutes or until aromatic.

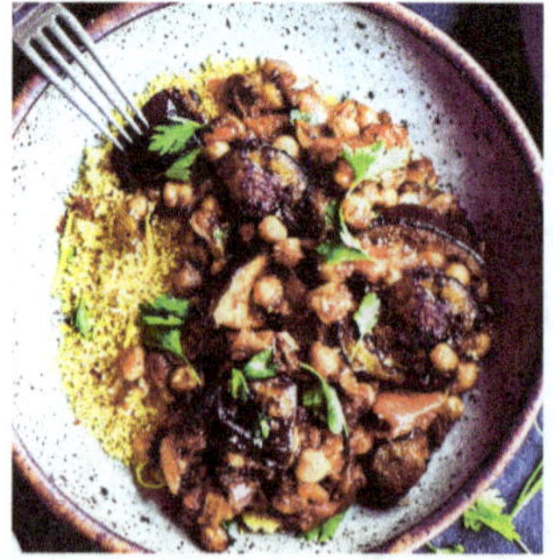

To the pan, add the drained chickpeas and diced tomatoes together with their liquids. Mix well to combine.

To taste, add salt and pepper for seasoning.

Once the aubergine is soft and the flavours have blended, cover the skillet or tagine and simmer the mixture over low heat for 20 to 25 minutes, stirring from time to time.

Taste after cooking and adjust seasoning *if needed.*

Serve the hot tagine of eggplant and chickpeas over cooked rice or couscous, topped with freshly chopped cilantro or parsley.

Spinach and Ricotta Stuffed Shells

Ingredients:

- One 12-oz package of large Pasta shells
- Two cups of cheese Ricotta
- 1 ½ cups finely chopped fresh spinach *(or thawed and drained frozen spinach)*
- One cup of finely shredded mozzarella cheese
- Grated Parmesan cheese, half a cup
- One egg, whisked just enough
- 2 minced garlic cloves
- One tsp of dehydrated oregano
- One tsp of dried basil
- Salt and pepper.
- 2 cups of marinara sauce

- Garnish with fresh basil leaves, *if desired.*

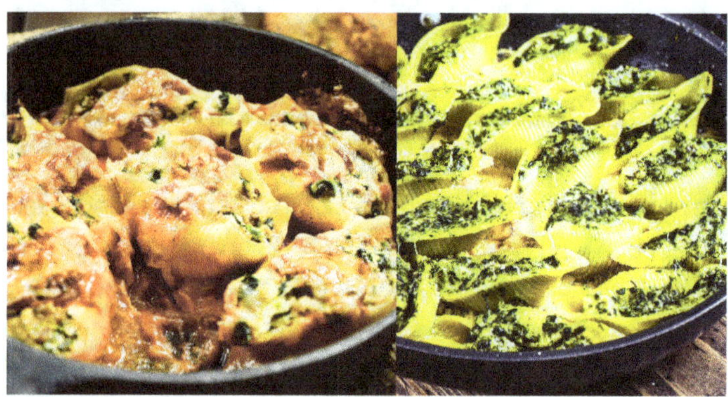

Instruction:

Set the oven temperature to 350°F (175°C). Grease and put aside a 9 x 13-inch baking dish.

As directed on the box, cook the giant pasta shells until they are al dente. After draining, let cool somewhat.

Ricotta cheese, chopped spinach, shredded mozzarella cheese, grated Parmesan cheese, egg, minced garlic, dried oregano, dried basil, salt and pepper should all be combined in a large mixing basin.

Stir well to include all of the ingredients.

Evenly distribute a large spoonful of marinara sauce on the bottom of the baking dish that has been prepared.

Using a spoon, carefully fill each cooked pasta shell with the spinach and ricotta filling. Top the marinara sauce-covered filled shells in the baking dish.

After stuffing each shell to capacity and arranging them in the baking dish, fill each shell entirely with a spoonful of the leftover marinara sauce.

Bake the dish in the preheated oven for 25 to 30 minutes or until the cheese is melted and bubbling and the shells are well cooked, covered with aluminium foil.

After removing the foil from the baking dish, bake the shells for a further 5 to 10 minutes or until the edges are beginning to become golden brown.

Before serving, take the filled shells out of the oven and let them cool for a few minutes.

If preferred, garnish with fresh basil leaves and serve hot.

Savour your mouth watering Stuffed Shells with Spinach and Ricotta. This dish can be customised.

Cauliflower Steak with Chimichurri Sauce

Ingredients:

For the Steak made with Cauliflower:

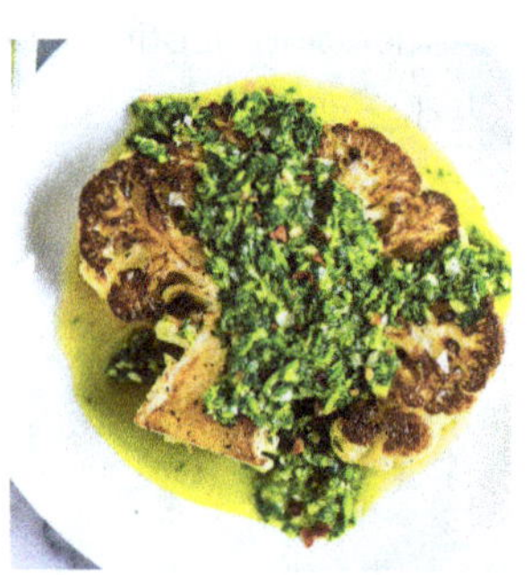

- One huge cauliflower head
- Two tsp olive oil
- Salt and pepper.

For the Sauce de Chimichurri:

- One cup of newly cut, freshly parsley
- 1/4 cup coarsely chopped fresh cilantro
- 3 minced garlic cloves
- One shallot, cut finely
- Half a cup of extra virgin olive oil
- 2 tsp red wine vinegar
- One tablespoon of lemon juice
- One tsp of dehydrated oregano
- Half a teaspoon of red pepper flakes, or to taste
- Salt and pepper.

Instruction:

Steak with Cauliflower: Set the oven temperature to 425°F (220°C).

Remove the cauliflower's stem and leaves, but do not cut the core.

Cut the cauliflower into pieces that are one inch thick, like "steaks."

Arrange the cauliflower steaks onto a parchment paper-lined baking sheet.

Season the cauliflower steaks to taste with salt and pepper after drizzling them with olive oil.

Roast the cauliflower for 25 to 30 minutes in a preheated oven or until it is soft and has a golden brown crust around the edges.

To make the chimichurri sauce - Place the chopped shallot, chopped parsley, chopped cilantro and minced garlic in a medium-sized bowl.

To the bowl, add the dried oregano, red pepper flakes, lemon juice, extra virgin olive oil and red wine vinegar.

To taste, add salt and pepper for seasoning and blend each component until well mixed. *If needed,* adjust the seasoning by tasting it.

Transfer the roasted cauliflower steaks to a plate for serving.

Drizzle the cauliflower steaks with a large amount of chimichurri sauce.

If desired, top hot dish with more chopped cilantro or parsley.

Black Bean and Corn Enchiladas

Ingredients:

Regarding the Enchilada filler:

- One can (15 oz) of rinsed and drained black beans
- One cup of fresh, canned or frozen Corn kernels
- One little onion, chopped
- One chopped bell pepper
- two minced garlic cloves
- One teaspoon of cumin powder
- One tsp of chilli powder
- Salt and pepper.
- One cup of grated cheese *(mixture of Monterey Jack, cheddar or blend)*
- 8 to 10 little corn tortillas or flour tortillas

For the Sauce on enchiladas:

- 2 tsp olive oil
- 2 tablespoons of flour (all-purpose)
- 2 tsp of chilli powder
- One teaspoon of cumin powder
- half a teaspoon of powdered garlic
- ¼ teaspoon of oregano, dried
- ¼ tsp salt
- Two cups of chicken or veggie broth

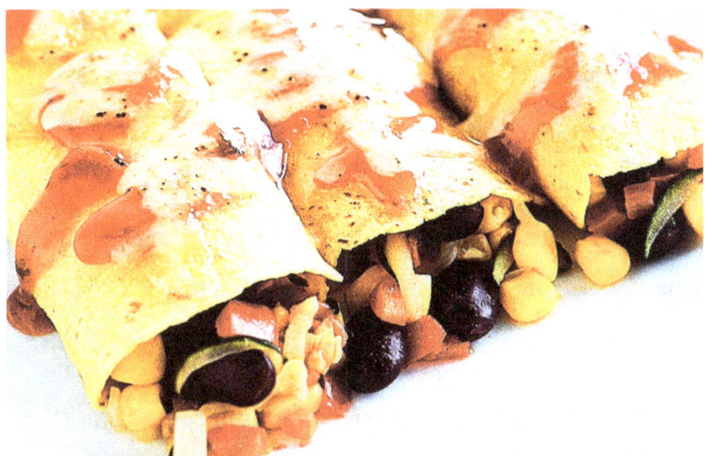

- **Extra toppings at your discretion:**
  chopped cilantro - fresh, Cut jalapeños, chopped
  avocado
  Greek yoghurt or sour cream

Instruction:

Turn the oven on to 375°F or 190°C. Set aside a baking dish that has been greased with cooking spray or olive oil.

Heat some olive oil in a big skillet over medium heat.

Saute the chopped onion and bell pepper for about 5 minutes or until they become tender.

Once aromatic, add the minced garlic, ground cumin, chilli powder, salt and pepper. Cook for an additional minute.

Add the corn kernels and black beans and stir. Cook for a few minutes or until well heated.

When well cooked, turn off the heat, set the skillet aside.

Heat the olive oil in a pot over medium heat to prepare the enchilada sauce. Stir in the salt, powdered cumin, dried oregano, garlic powder, chilli powder and flour. Stirring continually, cook for 1 to 2 minutes or until aromatic.

Stir in the veggie broth little by little until smooth. Simmer the sauce for 5 to 7 minutes, stirring now and again, until it thickens a little.

Take off the heat and put it aside.

Spoon a good portion of the black bean and corn mixture onto each tortilla, followed by the shredded cheese, to create the enchiladas.

After rolling the tortillas, put them seam-side down in the baking dish that has been ready.

Making careful to cover the prepared enchiladas equally, pour the enchilada sauce over them.

If you'd like, put more cheese on top.

Bake for 20 to 25 minutes in a preheated oven or until the cheese is bubbling and melted and the enchiladas are well cooked.

Take it out of the oven and let it cool down a little before serving.

Garnish the enchiladas with your preferred toppings, including diced avocado, sliced jalapeños and chopped cilantro.

Veggie Stir-Fry Noodles

Ingredients:

- 8 ounces or around 225 grams of noodles—such as soba, udon or rice noodles.
- 2 tsp of vegetable oil
- 2 minced garlic cloves
- One little onion, cut thinly
- One bell pepper, cut thinly
- One medium carrot, cut into thin slices or julienned
- one cup florets of broccoli
- One cup of sliced mushrooms, if desired
- One cup of snow peas or snap peas with the ends cut
- 2 teaspoons of soy sauce *(you may use tamari if you're gluten free)*
- One tablespoon of oyster sauce *(vegan option: use vegetarian oyster sauce)*
- One tablespoon of sesame oil
- One tsp finely chopped ginger *(optional)*
- Salt and pepper.
- **As a garnish,** add chopped green onions and sesame seeds (optional).

Instruction:

Noodles should be cooked as directed on the box until they are al dente. After draining, set aside.

Heat the vegetable oil in a big skillet or wok over medium-high heat.

Add the onion slices and minced garlic, and sauté for one to two minutes or until the onion starts to soften.

Snap peas, broccoli florets, sliced bell pepper, julienned carrot and mushrooms *(if used)* should all be added to the pan.

Stir-fry the veggies for 3–4 minutes or until they are crisp-tender.

Combine the soy sauce, oyster sauce, sesame oil and grated ginger *(if using)* in a small bowl. After adding the sauce to the veggies in the pan, stir to mix.

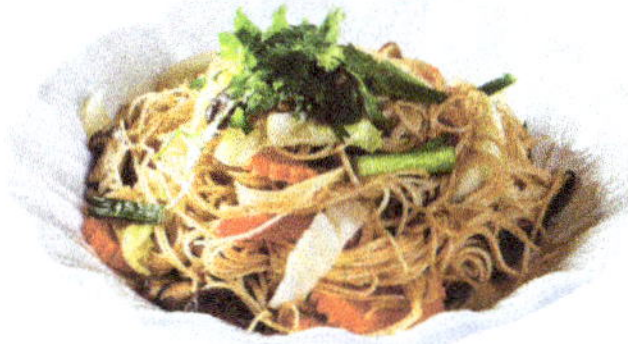

When the noodles are fully heated and thoroughly covered with sauce, add them to the pan and mix for 2 to 3 minutes.

If necessary, add more salt and pepper to the seasoning after tasting. **If preferred,** top the hot vegetable stir-fry noodles with chopped green onions and sesame seeds.

Creamy Mushroom Risotto

Ingredients:

- 1 ½ cups rice, Arborio
- 4 cups of chicken or veggie broth and one cup of dry white wine
- Two tsp olive oil
- two tsp butter
- One little onion, diced finely
- 8 ounces of sliced or cremini or button mushrooms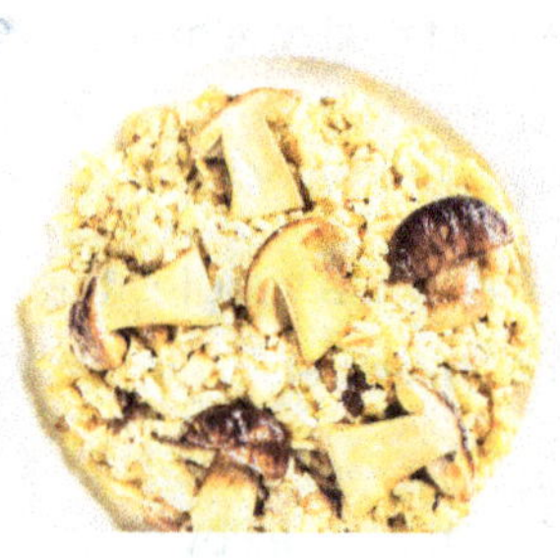
- 2 chopped garlic cloves
- Grated Parmesan cheese, half a cup
- Salt and pepper.
- Chopped fresh parsley *(for garnish)*
- **(Optional)** Truffle oil to drizzle

Instruction:

In a saucepan, heat the vegetable or chicken broth and maintain a low temperature.

Heat the butter and olive oil in a different, sizable skillet or saucepan over medium heat.

Add the chopped onion and garlic and cook for 3–4 minutes or until softened.

When the mushrooms are golden brown and soft, add the sliced ones to the pan and cook for 5 to 6 minutes.

To taste, add salt and pepper for seasoning.

Add the Arborio rice and cook, stirring frequently, for 1 to 2 minutes or until the rice is well covered with the oil and butter combination.

Add the white wine and stir continuously while cooking until the rice absorbs the liquid.

One ladleful at a time, add the heated broth to the rice mixture, stirring continuously and letting each addition soak in before adding more.

Continue cooking for another 18 to 20 minutes or until the rice is creamy and cooked through.

When the risotto reaches the consistency you want, toss in the grated Parmesan cheese and stir until it melts and is well mixed.

If needed, add more salt and pepper to the seasoning.

After turning off the heat, set aside the risotto to rest for a few minutes.

Serve hot, topped with freshly chopped parsley and, if preferred, a dab of truffle oil.

Spinach and Artichoke Stuffed Spaghetti Squash

Ingredients:

- One medium-sized spaghetti squash
- One tablespoon of olive oil
- 2 minced garlic cloves
- One little onion, chopped
- One 14-ounce can of drained and chopped artichoke hearts.
- 2 cups freshly chopped spinach
- Grated Parmesan cheese, ½ a cup
- ½ a cup of shredded mozzarella cheese
- Salt and pepper.
- Chopped fresh parsley *(for garnish)*

Instruction:

Set oven temperature to 400°F or 200°C.

Split the spaghetti squash in half lengthwise, then use a spoon to remove the seeds.

Arrange the halves on a baking sheet covered with parchment paper, cut side down.

The spaghetti squash should be baked for 40 to 50 minutes in a preheated oven or until the flesh is fork-tender.

Heat the olive oil in a big pan over medium heat while the squash bakes. Add the chopped onion and minced garlic and cook for 3–4 minutes or until the ingredients are soft and aromatic.

Cook the chopped spinach in the pan for 2 to 3 minutes or until it wilts.

Cook for a further 2 to 3 minutes after adding the chopped artichoke hearts.

After baking, take the spaghetti squash out of the oven and allow it to cool somewhat. Using a fork, scrape the squash's flesh into strands, leaving a 1/4-inch border all the way around.

After transferring the spaghetti squash strands, add the spinach and artichoke mixture to the pan. Add the grated Parmesan cheese - taste and adjust the seasoning.

Evenly divide the mixture between the two sides of the spaghetti squash, pressing it down a little.

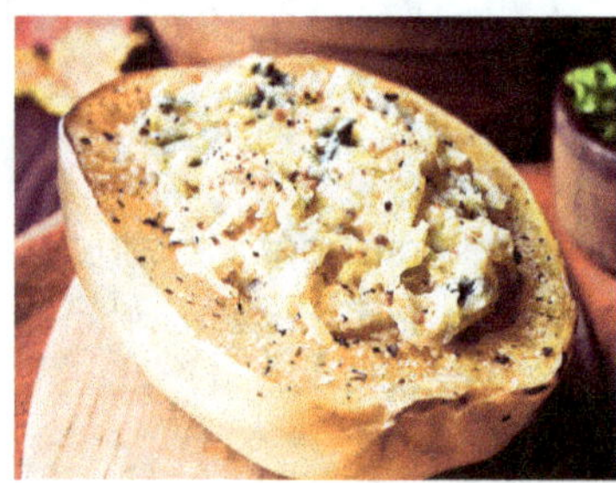

Top each packed squash half with shredded mozzarella cheese.

Put the packed squash halves back in the oven and continue to bake for 10 to 15 more minutes or until the cheese is bubbling and melted.

When the squash is cooked, take it out of the oven and top it with freshly cut parsley before serving.

Lentil Shepherd's Pie

Ingredients:

Regarding the Lentil stuffing:

- One cup of washed and dried green or brown lentils
- Three cups of vegetable broth
- One tablespoon of olive oil
- One sliced onion
- 2 chopped carrots
- 2 minced garlic cloves
- A single tsp of dried thyme
- One tsp of dehydrated rosemary
- One tsp of paprika
- Salt and pepper.
- One cup of frozen peas

Regarding the Mashed Potato garnish:

- 4 big potatoes, chopped and skinned
- 1/4 cup non dairy milk - such oat or almond milk
- Two teaspoons of olive oil or vegan butter
- Salt and pepper.

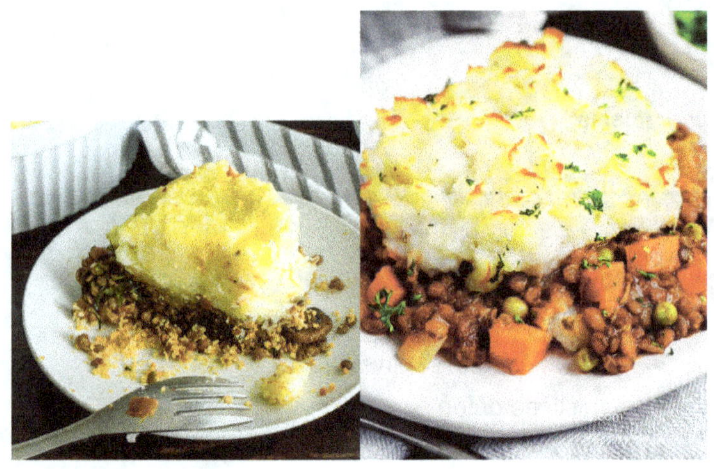

Instructions:

Turn the oven on to 375°F, or 190°C.

Combine the lentils and vegetable broth in a large pot. Once the lentils are soft and the majority of the liquid has been absorbed, bring to a boil, then lower the heat to a simmer for 20 to 25 minutes.

Make the mashed potatoes while the lentils are cooking.

In a large saucepan of water, add the diced potatoes and bring to a boil. Simmer for 15 to 20 minutes or until the potatoes are fork-tender. After draining, put the potatoes back in the saucepan.

Use a fork or potato masher to mash the potatoes. Once the vegan butter or olive oil, non dairy milk, salt and pepper are added, mash until smooth and creamy. Set aside.

Heat the olive oil in a big skillet over medium heat. Cook the chopped onion and carrots for 5 to 7 minutes or until they are tender.

Cook for a further 2 minutes after adding the minced garlic, paprika, dried thyme, dried rosemary, salt and pepper.

Toss in the frozen peas and cooked lentils with the veggies in the pan. Cook, stirring, for a further 2 to 3 minutes or until the peas are well heated.

Spread the lentil mixture evenly in a 9 by 13-inch baking dish after transferring it there. Spread out the mashed potatoes into an equal layer on top of the lentil mixture using a spoon.

After preheating the oven, place the baking dish inside and bake for 25 to 30 minutes or until the mixture is bubbling around the edges and the mashed potatoes are golden brown.

Before serving, take out of the oven and let it cool for a few minutes.

Savour your Shepherd's Pie with Lentil.

Veggie Tikka Masala with Basmati Rice

Ingredients:

For the Tikka Masala with Veggies:

- Two cups of mixed veggies, including peas, carrots, cauliflower and bell peppers
- One cup of plain yoghurt *(for a vegan variation, use dairy-free yoghurt)*
- 2 tsp of the tikka masala spice mixture
- 2 tsp of vegetable oil
- One onion, chopped finely
- 3 chopped garlic cloves, one inch of grated ginger
- 1 can or 14 ounces chopped tomatoes
- Half a cup of coconut milk
- One cup of vegetable broth
- Add salt to taste.

- **To garnish,** use fresh cilantro leaves.

Regarding the Basmati Rice:

- One cup of rice, basmati
- two cups of water
- Add salt to taste.

Instruction:

Chop the veggies into small pieces to prepare them.

Combine the yoghurt and tikka masala spice blend in a bowl and stir until well mixed.

After adding the mixed veggies to the dish, swirl them around to ensure the marinade coats them evenly.

For optimal flavour, marinate it for at least half an hour, preferably overnight in the refrigerator.

Rinse the basmati rice under cold water until the water runs clear while the veggies are marinating.

This aids in removing too much starch. Next, combine the rice with two cups of water and a little amount of salt in a saucepan. After bringing to a boil, lower the heat to a simmer, cover and allow the rice to cook for 15 to 20 minutes or until it is fluffy.

In a big skillet, warm the vegetable oil over medium heat.

Add the chopped onion and sauté for 5 to 7 minutes or until it is tender and transparent.

Cook for a further 1 to 2 minutes or until aromatic, after adding the grated ginger and minced garlic.

When the veggies are somewhat soft, add the marinated ones to the pan and simmer, turning periodically, for approximately 5 to 7 minutes.

After adding the vegetable broth and chopped tomatoes, mix everything together. Once the mixture reaches a simmer, cook it for a further 10 to 15 minutes, so that the flavours can combine and the sauce may gradually thicken.

After adding the coconut milk, taste and add salt as needed. Give it five more minutes to boil.

Serve the hot Veggie Tikka Masala over the prepared basmati rice as soon as it's done. Before serving, garnish with fresh cilantro leaves.

Grilled Vegetable Skewers with Quinoa Pilaf

Ingredients:

For the Skewers of Grilled Vegetables:

- One sliced courgette
- One sliced yellow squash
- Cut one red bell pepper into pieces.
- One green bell pepper that has been diced
- One red onion, sliced into pieces
- Rosy tomatoes
- Water-soaked wooden skewers, soaking for at least half an hour

Regarding the Marinade:

- 1 ¼ cup olive oil
- 2 minced garlic cloves
- Half a tsp balsamic vinegar
- One tsp of dehydrated oregano
- Salt and pepper.

For the Pilaf with Quinoa:

- One cup of washed quinoa
- 2 cups water or vegetable broth
- One tablespoon of olive oil
- One little onion, chopped
- 2 minced garlic cloves
- half a cup of carrots, chopped
- Half a cup of chopped bell pepper, any colour
- half a cup of frozen peas
- Salt and pepper.
- Chopped fresh parsley **(for garnish)**

Instructions:

Set your grill's temperature to medium-high.

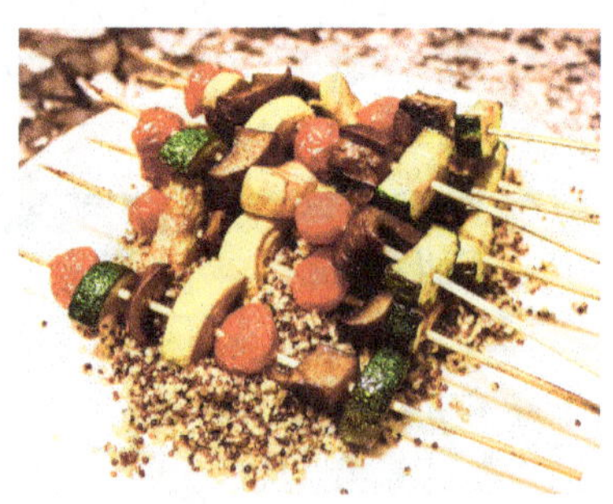

Combine all of the marinade's ingredients in a small bowl.

As desired, thread the cut veggies in a thread pattern onto the moistened skewers. After arranging the skewers in a shallow dish, coat the veggies with marinade.

Give them 10 to 15 minutes to marinade.

Make the quinoa pilaf while the veggies are marinating.

Heat the olive oil in a saucepan over medium heat. Add the chopped onion and simmer for 3–4 minutes or until transparent. Add the minced garlic and continue cooking for one more minute.

Stirring constantly, add the quinoa to the pot and toast it for 2 to 3 minutes.

Add the water or veggie broth and heat until it boils.

After lowering the heat, cover and let simmer the quinoa for 15 to 20 minutes - it should be cooked and fluffy.

Heat a little amount of olive oil in a different pan over medium heat and cook for 5 to 7 minutes or until the bell pepper and chopped carrots are starting to soften.

Add the frozen peas and simmer for a further 2 to 3 minutes.

To taste, add salt and pepper for seasoning.

After the quinoa is done, add the sautéed veggies and fluff it with a fork. To stay warm, remove from the heat and cover.

As the quinoa cooks, grill the vegetable skewers for 8 to 10 minutes, rotating them from time to time, until the veggies become soft and slightly browned.

Serve the quinoa pilaf with the grilled veggie skewers on the side. **If preferred**, garnish with finely chopped fresh parsley.

You can modify the spice and veggies to suit your tastes.

SNACKS OPTIONS

Hummus and Veggie Sticks

Ingredients:

- 15 ounces *(one can)* of rinsed and drained chickpeas
- 2 to 3 tablespoons tahini or sesame paste
- 1 or 2 minced garlic cloves *(adjust to taste)*
- 2 to 3 teaspoons freshly squeezed lemon juice
- 2 to 3 tsp extra virgin olive oil
- Salt to taste.
- Water *(to change the consistency)*

- Various veggies *(carrots, cucumbers, bell peppers, celery, etc.)* for dipping

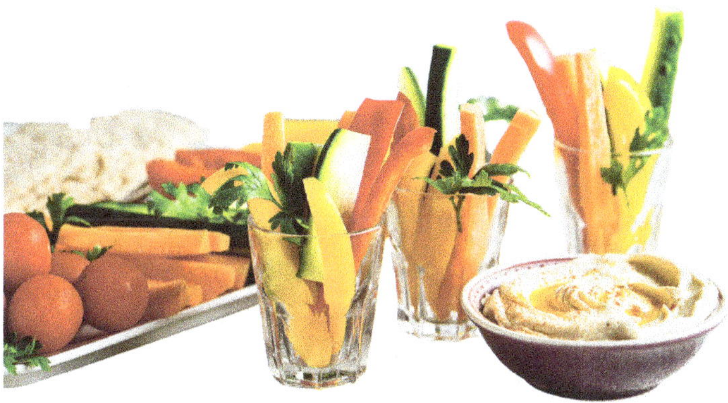

Instruction:

Give the chickpeas a good rinse in cold water. Make sure to thoroughly drain them.

Process the chickpeas, tahini, olive oil, lemon juice, chopped garlic and a dash of salt in a food processor. Process till smooth.

To get the right consistency, add a spoonful at a time of water if the hummus is too thick.

Taste the hummus and adjust the spices according to your preference. Depending on your taste, you may add more garlic, lemon juice or salt.

To serve, move the hummus into a bowl. Arrange the sticks of vegetables *(carrots, bell peppers, cucumbers, celery, etc.)* in a circle around the bowl.

Optional garnish: Drizzle a little more olive oil over the hummus. For added taste and appearance, you may also add some chopped fresh herbs or paprika.

Enjoy your homemade hummus and vegetable sticks right away after serving.

To make inventive hummus variants, try experimenting with other ingredients like sun-dried tomatoes, roasted red peppers or herbs like cilantro or parsley.

Trail Mix with Nuts and Dried Fruits

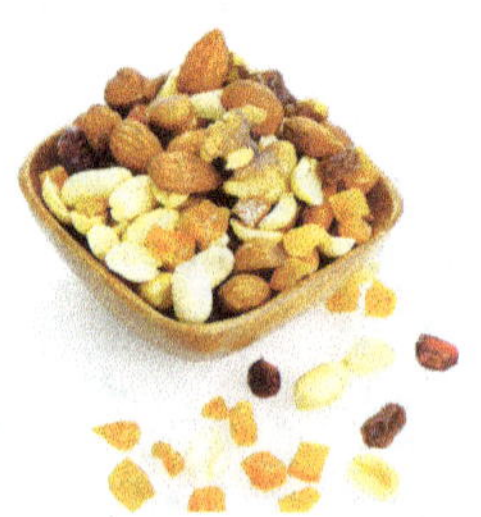

Ingredients:

- One cup of almonds
- One cup cashews

- One cup of peanuts
- 1 cup of cranberries, dried
- one cup of raisins
- ½ a cup of pumpkin seeds
- ½ a cup of sunflower seeds
- chopped half a cup of dried apricots
- ½ a cup of dried cherries
- ½ a cup of chocolate chips, if desired

Instruction:

Set the oven temperature to 350°F (175°C).

Arrange the cashews, almonds, peanuts, sunflower and pumpkin seeds on a baking sheet.

For approximately 8 to 10 minutes or until they are aromatic and softly golden brown, roast the nuts and seeds in the oven.

To avoid burning them, keep a watch on them.

After taking the baking sheet out of the oven, let the nuts and seeds cool fully.

Add the dried cranberries, raisins, dried apricots, dried cherries and chocolate chips *(if using)* to a large mixing bowl along with the cooled nuts and seeds.

Mix everything until well incorporated.

To store the trail mix, move it to a sealed receptacle or separate snack bags. Savour your own trail mix as a quick and healthful on-the-go snack.

Baked Kale Chips

A tasty and nutritious substitute for regular potato chips are baked kale chips. They are nutrient-dense, tasty and crispy.

Ingredients:

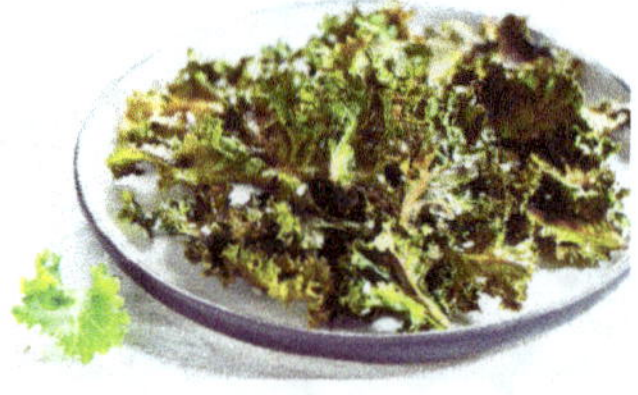

- 1 bunch of kale
- 1 or 2 teaspoons olive oil
- Add salt *(to taste)*.

- *Additions of optional spices* include nutritional yeast, chilli powder, paprika, onion powder and garlic powder.

Instruction:

Set the oven temperature to 350°F (175°C).

Get the kale ready: After giving the kale a good wash, cut off the stems.

Tear the leaves into small pieces, about 1 mouthful. Before moving forward, make sure they are entirely dry.

Toss the kale pieces in olive oil in a big dish. Just enough oil is needed to gently cover the leaves.

To guarantee a uniform coating, use your hands to gently massage the oil into the leaves.

For Seasoning: Toss the kale with salt and any other ingredients you'd like. For an even coat, toss.

Arrange the kale pieces on a baking sheet in a single layer. To guarantee consistent cooking, make sure they are not overlapping.

Bake for 10 to 15 minutes or until the kale is crispy and has a hint of colour around the edges. *They may burn rapidly, so keep an eye on them.*

Before serving, take the kale chips out of the oven and allow them to cool for a few minutes. Savour them as a side dish or as a snack.

Although leftover kale chips are best eaten fresh, you may keep them in an airtight container for up to several days. Just be advised that over time, they could get less crispy.

Avocado Slices on Whole Grain Crackers

Ingredients:

- Ripe avocados
- Crackers made entirely of grains
- Salt and pepper.
- Cherry tomatoes, cucumber slices, feta cheese, red pepper flakes, lime juice and other toppings *are optional.*

Instruction:

Cut the avocados in half and remove the pits first.

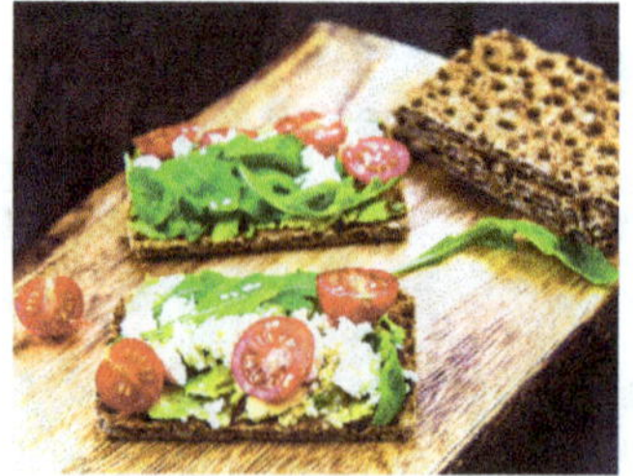

Scoop the avocado flesh into a bowl using a spoon. Using a fork, mash the avocado until the appropriate consistency is achieved. *Depending on your desire, you may either make it smooth or leave it somewhat lumpy.*

Add salt and pepper to taste while seasoning the mashed avocado. **If preferred,** you may also add a squeeze of lime juice for additional flavour.

Evenly distribute the mashed avocado over the whole grain crackers.

Add other toppings to the avocado spread if you'd like - such as cucumber slices, cherry tomatoes, crumbled feta cheese or a dash of red pepper flakes for spiciness.

Serve your avocado slices on whole grain crackers as a delicious and healthy snack or appetiser right away.

You can alter this recipe to suit your dietary needs and taste preferences.

Apple Slices with Peanut Butter

Ingredients:

- 1 or 2 apples of whatever kind you want
- Peanut butter *(choice of texture: smooth or crunchy)*
- Granola, honey, cinnamon, raisins, chopped almonds, and/or raisins are **optional toppings.**

Instruction:

After giving the apples a good wash under running water, blot dry with a fresh kitchen towel.

After removing the seeds and sections, core the apples and cut them into thin rounds or wedges.

Put a liberal dollop of peanut butter on each piece of apple.

To achieve this, you may use a spoon or butter knife.

Sprinkle some cinnamon on top for more flavour or pour some honey over the peanut butter for more sweetness, *if you'd like.*

Optional: Sprinkle granola, chopped almonds or raisins over the peanut butter.

Serve the apple slices right away after arranging them on a tray or serving dish.

Roasted Chickpeas with Spices

Ingredients:

- Two cans *(15 ounces each)* of washed and drained garbanzo beans or chickpeas.
- Two tsp olive oil
- One teaspoon of cumin powder
- One tsp of paprika
- ½ a teaspoon of powdered garlic
- ½ a teaspoon of powdered onion
- ¼ tsp cayenne *(adjust according to taste)*
- Salt to taste.
- **Optional:** freshly ground pepper granules

Instruction:

Set oven temperature to 400°F or 200°C.

After fully draining, give the chickpeas a thorough rinse in cold water. Using paper towels or a fresh kitchen towel, pat them dry.

They will crisp up more evenly in the oven if the extra moisture is removed.

Toss the dry chickpeas with olive oil in a big basin until they are well covered.

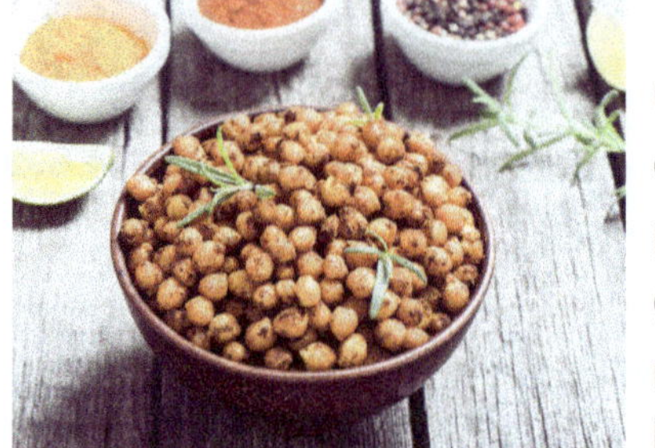

Combine the ground cumin, paprika, cayenne pepper, onion powder, garlic powder and black pepper, *if using,* in a small bowl.

Once the chickpeas are equally covered with spices, sprinkle the spice combination over them and toss.

Arrange the seasoned chickpeas in a single layer on an aluminium foil or parchment paper-lined baking sheet.

Bake for 25 to 35 minutes in a preheated oven, shaking or tossing the pan halfway through or until the chickpeas become crispy and golden brown.

After roasting, take the chickpeas out of the oven and allow them to cool down for a little while before serving. Eat the roasted chickpeas as an on-the-go crispy snack or as a garnish for grain bowls, salads and soups.

You may experiment with the spices to suit your tastes, varying the amount of cayenne pepper for spiciness or the amount of salt.

Rice Cakes with Almond Butter

Ingredients:

- Rice cakes *(As many as you'd like)*
- Almond butter
- **Optional Toppings include** shredded coconut, chia seeds, honey, sliced bananas and berries.

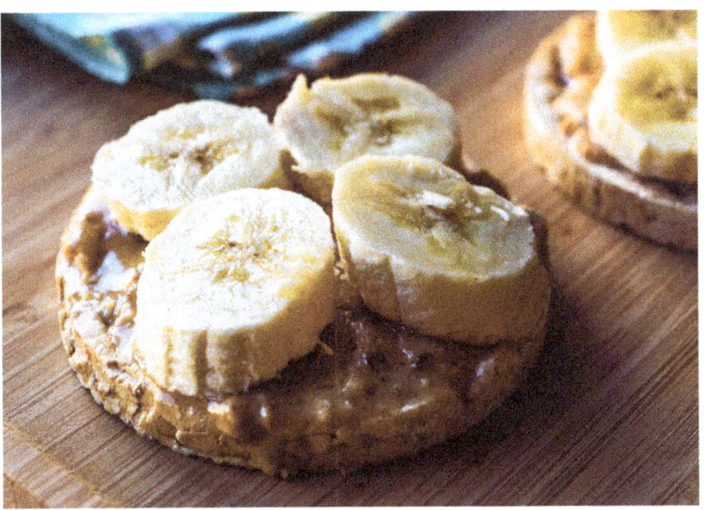

Instruction:

Spread a thick layer of almond butter over the top of a rice cake. You may choose almond butter that is crunchy or smooth, based on your taste.

For extra taste and nutrients, you may sprinkle shredded coconut, chia seeds, honey, banana slices or berries on top of the almond butter.

Continue this to make your desired amount of rice cakes.

Serve and savour as a light supper or a fast and healthful snack.You may alter this recipe to suit your dietary needs and tastes. If you'd rather try anything other than almond butter, feel free to experiment with other nut or seed butters.

Cucumber Slices with Cream Cheese and Dill

Ingredients:

- One huge cucumber
- Four ounces of softened cream cheese
- 1-2 teaspoons finely chopped fresh dill
- Salt and pepper.
- Zest of lemon, *if desired,* for added flavour

Instruction:

After giving the cucumber a good wash, blot it dry using paper towels.

Cut the cucumber into rounds that are thin and 1/4 inch thick.

The skin may be peeled *if you'd like,* or left on for more texture and colour.

Combine the melted cream cheese and finely chopped fresh dill in a small bowl, mixing them well. To taste, add salt and pepper for seasoning.

Add a little lemon zest if you want it to taste zesty.

Spoon a little bit of the cream cheese mixture onto each slice of cucumber, covering the whole surface.

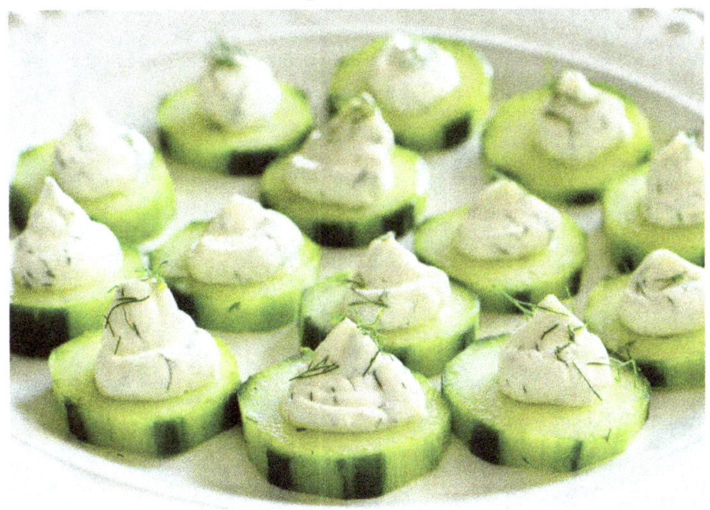

Place the cucumber slices on a dish or plate for serving. **If desired,** garnish with more lemon zest or dill.

Serve right away or put in the fridge until you're ready to serve. For any occasion, these cucumber slices with cream cheese and dill make a sophisticated and refreshing appetiser or snack.

Guacamole with Baked Tortilla Chips

Guacamole Ingredients:

- Two ripe avocados
- One little red onion, cut finely
- One or two chopped tomatoes
- Finely chopped and seeded jalapeño pepper *(optional; adjust to taste)*
- 2 minced garlic cloves
- 1 lime's juice
- Salt and pepper.
- Chop some fresh cilantro *(optional).*

Tortilla Chips Ingredients:

corn tortillas *(make whatever many you like)*
Cooking spray or olive oil

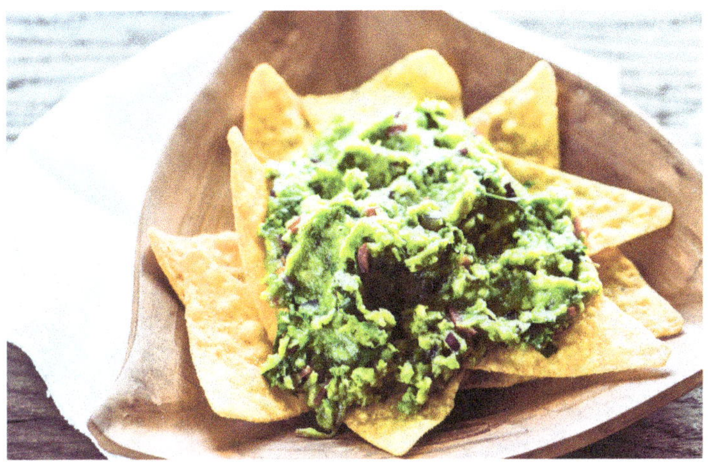

Instructions:

To begin, prepare the guacamole by cutting the avocados in half, removing the pits and transferring the flesh into a dish for mixing.

Using a fork, mash the avocados until you get the consistency you want *(some people like theirs chunkier, others smoother)*.

Chopped red onion, diced tomatoes, minced garlic, minced jalapeño *(if used)*, lime juice, salt, pepper and chopped cilantro *(if using)* should be added.

Toss to blend thoroughly.

Taste and, *if needed,* adjust seasoning. Depending on your taste, you may add more pepper, salt or lime juice.

Prepare the Tortilla Chips Baked:
Set the oven temperature to 175°C or 350°F.

Lightly apply cooking spray or a thin coat of olive oil on both sides of each corn tortilla.

Arrange the tortillas in a stack and cut them into wedges, just as you would a pizza.

Spread out the tortilla wedges on a baking sheet in a single layer. Verify that they do not overlap.

Lightly season the tortilla wedges with salt.

Bake the chips for 10 to 15 minutes or until they are crisp and golden. *Watch them closely since oven temperatures might change.*

Take out the crispy, cooked tortilla chips from the oven and let them cool slightly.

Serve the cooked tortilla chips with the guacamole, ready for dipping.

Energy Balls with Dates and Nuts

Nut and date energy balls are a delicious and nutritious snack choice. They don't need to be baked and are simple to create.

Ingredients:

- 1 cup of dates, pitted
- One cup of your preferred nuts, such as cashews, walnuts, almonds or a combination
- One-fourth cup rolled oats
- One tablespoon of **optional** chia seeds
- One tablespoon of **optional** flaxseed meal
- One teaspoon of **optional** vanilla extract
- A dash of salt
- *Other choices for coating include* chopped almonds, hemp hearts, cocoa powder, shredded coconut and sesame seeds *(optional)*.

Instruction:

Immerse the Dates: To soften dates that are dry, immerse them in warm water for 10 to 15 minutes.

To prepare the nuts, either coarsely chop them by hand or pulse them several times in a food processor until they are finely chopped if you are using whole nuts. Take care not to overprocess or you may turn your food into nut butter.

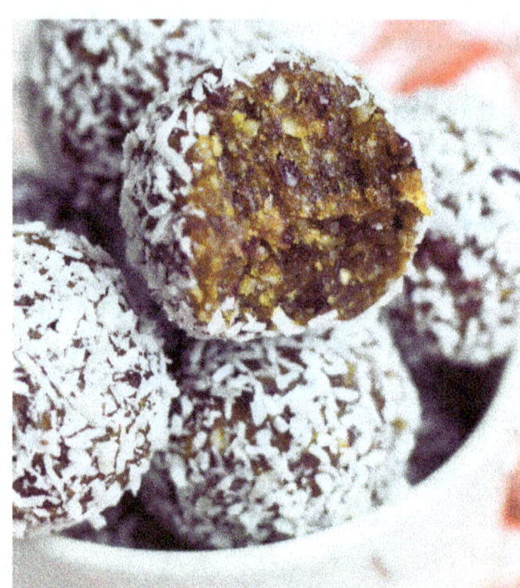

Place the drained and soaked dates, chopped almonds, rolled oats, chia seeds, flaxseed meal, vanilla extract *(if using)*, and a dash of salt in a food processor.

Mix the ingredients until a sticky dough begins to form, about 30 seconds. You may add additional dates or a teaspoon or two of water if it's too dry.

Create Balls: Using little amounts of the mixture, roll them between your hands to create tiny balls that have a diameter of approximately an inch. *You may moisten your hands with water to keep your hands from adhering if the mixture is too sticky to manage.*

Coat the Balls (Optional): For added taste and texture, roll the balls in chopped almonds, hemp hearts, sesame seeds, shredded coconut or cocoa powder.

Adapting the coatings to your own tastes allows you to become creative.

To make the energy balls firmer, place them on a plate or baking sheet covered with parchment paper and refrigerate for at least ½ an hour.

Storage: The energy balls may be kept in the refrigerator for up to 2 weeks once they have been cooled.

Simply move them to an airtight container. Moreover, they may be frozen for extended storage.

When you need a fast snack or an energy boost before a workout, try these tasty and nourishing energy balls. You can modify the ingredients and amounts to suit your dietary needs and personal tastes.

Green Smoothie with Spinach, Banana and Almond Milk

Ingredients:

- One ripe banana
- One cup of raw spinach
- One cup almond milk *(you may substitute any other kind of milk)*
- **Optional:** For sweetness, use one spoonful of honey or maple syrup.
- For a cooler smoothie - Add 1/2 cup of ice cubes *optionally.*

Instruction:

After peeling, chop the banana into little pieces.

Thoroughly wash the spinach leaves.

Blend the spinach leaves, banana pieces, almond milk and sugar *(if used)* in a blender.

To make the smoothie cooler, feel free to add ice cubes.

Mix every item until it becomes creamy and smooth.

You may adjust the consistency by adding more almond milk if it's too thick.

After tasting the smoothie, add additional honey or maple syrup *if needed* to make it more sweet.

After transferring the smoothie into glasses, serve it right away.

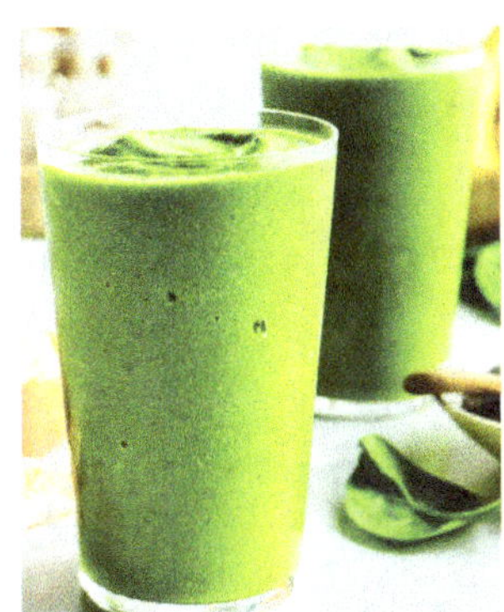

Berry Blast Smoothie with Mixed Berries and Greek Yoghurt

Ingredients:

- One cup of mixed berries *(blackberries, raspberries, blueberries and strawberries)*
- Half a cup of plain or vanilla-flavoured Greek yoghurt
- Half a cup of milk *(vegan or non-vegan).*
- One tablespoon of maple syrup or honey *(optional; adds sweetness)*
- **(Optional, for a cooler smoothie)** Ice cubes

Instruction:

The mixed berries should be well cleaned under running water and then patted dry with paper towels.

Remove the stems off strawberries *if using them*.

In a blender, combine the mixed berries, Greek yoghurt, milk and honey or maple syrup *(if desired)*.

You may also add a few ice cubes if you'd like your smoothie to be cooler.

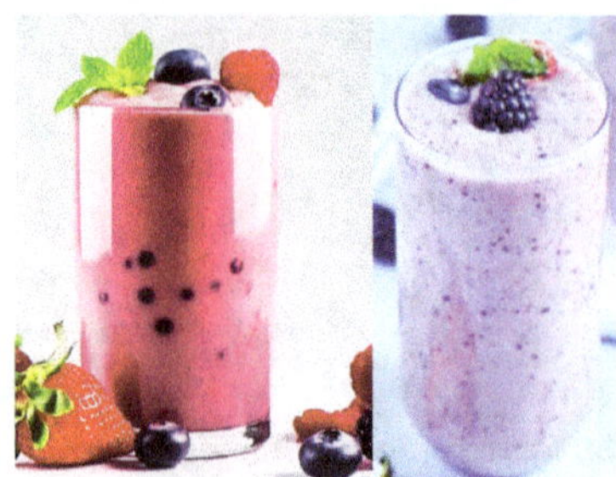

Combine all ingredients in a blender and process until smooth and creamy. You may add extra milk if the consistency is too thick to get the right thickness.

After tasting the smoothie, add additional honey or maple syrup ***if needed*** to make it more sweet.

When you are done blending to your desired consistency, transfer the smoothie into glasses and serve right away. If you'd like, you may add more berries or a sprig of mint to the smoothie for presentation.

Tropical Paradise Smoothie with Mango, Pineapple and Coconut Milk

Ingredients:

- One ripe mango, chopped and peeled
- 1 cup of frozen or fresh Pineapple chunks
- One cup of coconut milk *(either carton or canned)*
- Half a cup of ice cubes
- **If desired,** add honey or agave syrup for sweetness.

Instruction:

Start by getting your ingredients ready. If using fresh pineapple, slice it into bits and peel and cube the mango.

You may omit this step if your pineapple is frozen.

Place the chopped mango, pieces of pineapple, coconut milk and ice cubes into a blender.

Optional: At this point, you may choose to sprinkle in some honey or agave syrup if you'd like your smoothie to be sweeter.

Combine all ingredients in a blender and process until smooth and creamy. You may adjust the consistency by adding more coconut milk or a little amount of water if it's too thick.

After the smoothie is blended to your desired consistency,

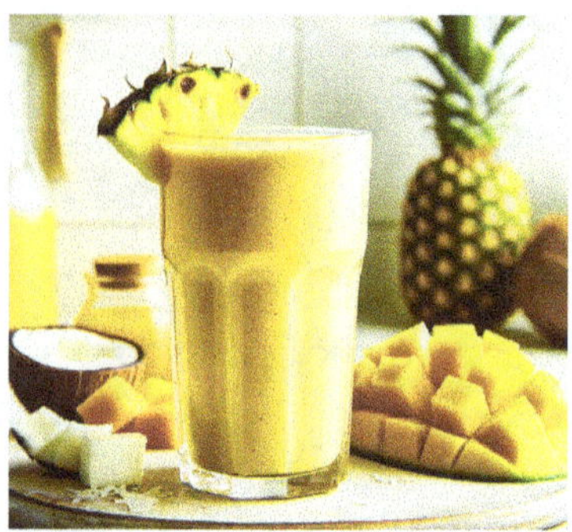 taste it and add additional honey or agave syrup to modify the sweetness *if needed.*

After transferring the smoothie into glasses, serve it right away.

If you would like, you may add more mango or pineapple slices as a garnish for an even more tropical flair.

It's ok to modify the amounts of each fruit and coconut milk to suit your own taste preferences. For further taste variations, you can also alter this recipe by using other tropical fruits like papaya or banana.

Chocolate Peanut Butter Smoothie with Protein Powder

Ingredients:

- 1 frozen ripe banana
- One tsp unsweetened chocolate powder

- One spoonful of sugar-free, natural peanut butter
- One scoop of protein powder with chocolate flavour
- One cup of unsweetened almond milk or any other kind of milk you like.
- Greek yoghurt, 1/2 cup *(optional; adds creaminess)*
- **(Optional, for a richer smoothie)** ice cubes

Instruction:

After peeling, chop the banana into large pieces. To give the smoothie a cooler texture later on, feel free to add some ice cubes if it's not frozen.

Blend together the protein powder, peanut butter, chocolate, frozen banana chunks, almond milk and Greek yoghurt *(if desired)* in a blender.

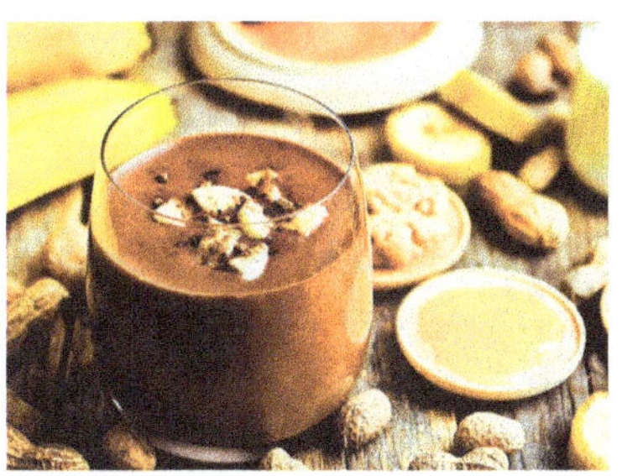

Mix every item until it becomes creamy and smooth.

You may adjust the consistency by adding a little extra almond milk if it's too thick.

Taste the smoothie and add additional cocoa powder,

peanut butter or sweetener **if needed** to modify the sweetness or thickness.

After everything has been well mixed and smooth, serve the smoothie right away by pouring it into glasses.

For added taste and visual appeal, you may optionally top the smoothie with chopped peanuts, chocolate powder or more peanut butter drizzled over it.

Beetroot and Berry Smoothie with Flax Seeds

Ingredients:

- 1/2 cup mixed berries *(strawberries, raspberries and blueberries)*
- 1 small peeled and diced beetroot
- One ripe banana, cut into slices and peeled
- One spoonful of Flax seeds
- Half a cup of plain yoghurt or vegan-friendly dairy-free yoghurt
- Half a cup of almond milk or any other kind of milk you like
- One tablespoon of honey or maple syrup *(optional, depending on desired level of sweetness)*
- Ice cubes *(optional, if you want your smoothie cooler)*

Instruction:

Get the ingredients ready: Beetroot should be cleaned and cut into tiny pieces. Slice and peel the banana and rinse your berries well if they are fresh.

Put the diced beets, mixed berries, banana slices, flax seeds, plain yoghurt, almond milk and, *if desired,* honey or maple syrup in a blender.

Process the ingredients in a blender until a creamy, smooth consistency is reached. Add more yoghurt or banana to make your smoothie thicker if that's your preference.

You may thin down a thick smoothie by adding more almond milk. Also add ice cubes if it's too thin, then mix it once more to get the right consistency.

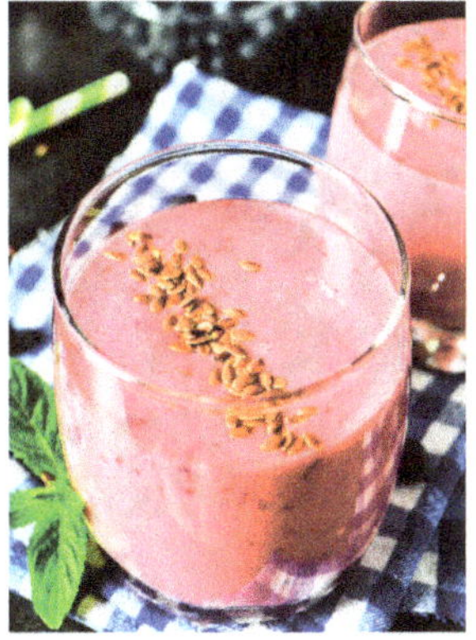

If necessary, add additional honey or maple syrup to the smoothie to make it more sweet.

Immediately serve the smoothie by pouring it into glasses. **If preferred,** you may top with a sprinkling of flax seeds or a few more berries as a garnish.

Cucumber Mint Cooler

Ingredients:

- One chopped and peeled cucumber
- 1 ¼ cup of fresh mint leaves
- 2 tsp lemon juice
- 2 teaspoons of sugar or honey, according to taste
- 2 glasses of cold water
- Cucumber slices and mint sprigs **as garnish** on ice cubes

Instruction:

Cucumber, mint leaves, lemon juice, honey or sugar and cold water should all be combined in a blender.

Blend until thoroughly integrated and smooth.

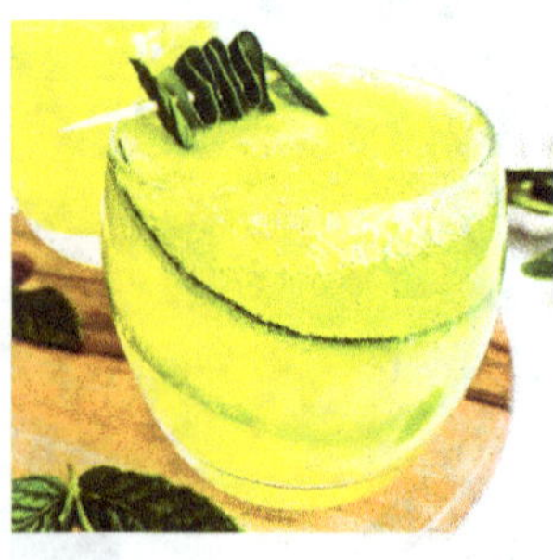

If necessary, taste the mixture and add additional honey, sugar or lemon juice to adjust the sweetness or sharpness.

To get rid of any pulp or seeds, strain the mixture using

cheesecloth or a fine mesh screen - *you may skip this step if you'd want your texture to be smoother.*

Place ice cubes in serving glasses and fill the cups with the cucumber-mint mixture.

Add cucumber slices and sprigs of mint as garnish.

Enjoy your cool Cucumber Mint Cooler right away.

You can change the ingredients to suit your tastes. This drink may also be made fizzy by adding a dash of soda or sparkling water.

Watermelon Basil Refresher

For hot summer days, the pleasant and cool Watermelon Basil Refresher is ideal.

Ingredients:

- 4 cups of freshly cut, seeded watermelon pieces
- 1/4 cup finely chopped fresh basil leaves
- Two tablespoons *(or more, depending on taste)* of honey or agave syrup
- 1 lime's juice
- 2 glasses of chilled water

- Cubes of ice
- Garnish with watermelon slices and basil leaves *(optional).*

Instruction:

Get the basil and watermelon ready:

Make sure all the seeds are out before chopping the watermelon into bits.

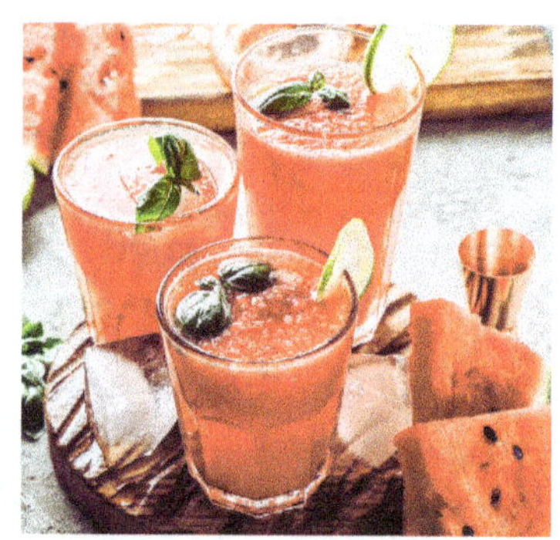

After giving the basil leaves a good rinse, finely cut them and mix basil with watermelon pieces to a blender.

Process till smooth.

Optional: To get a smoother consistency, you may remove any pulp from the blended mixture by straining it through a fine mesh screen.

Transfer the combined combination of watermelon and basil into a pitcher.

As needed - sweetness may be adjusted by adding honey or agave syrup.

To add some tang, squeeze in the juice of one lime. Depending on how much lime juice you desire, adjust the quantity and pour in some cold water.

To dilute the mixture and get the desired consistency, stir in the cold water.

Put the pitcher in the fridge to cool for half an hour or longer.

When ready to serve, place ice cubes in glasses and top with cooled Watermelon Basil Refresher.

For a pretty touch, place a little slice of watermelon or a basil leaf on the rim of each glass.

Before pouring, give the drink a little stir to make sure all the flavours are incorporated, then serve.

Change the ingredients to suit your tastes. You may adjust the flavour to your preference by experimenting with different herbs or fruits.

Golden Milk with Turmeric and Ginger

In Ayurvedic tradition, golden milk - sometimes called turmeric milk or turmeric latte, is a warming and soothing drink that has been enjoyed for millennia.

Ingredients:

- Two cups of milk *(you may use whatever kind of milk you choose, such oat, almond, coconut or cow's milk)*
- 1 tsp finely ground turmeric
- 1 teaspoon of fresh ginger, coarsely grated or half a teaspoon of ground ginger.
- One tablespoon of maple syrup or honey, adjusted to taste
- 1/4 tsp ground cinnamon *(may be added).*
- A little amount of black pepper *(which improves turmeric absorption)*

Instruction:

Heat the milk in a small saucepan over medium heat.

Stir the ground turmeric, fresh or ground ginger, honey, maple syrup and, *if desired,* cinnamon into the milk.

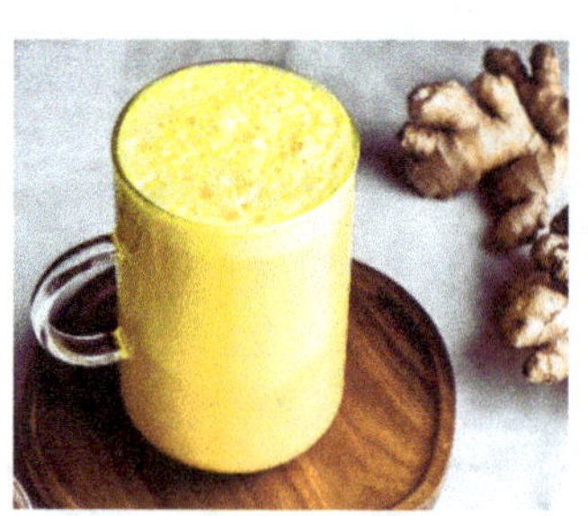

Mix well to blend.

Simmer the liquid slowly for around 5 minutes, stirring from time to time.

After taking the pot from the stove, let the golden milk cool somewhat.

If using fresh ginger, strain the golden milk through a fine-mesh screen to get rid of any pieces of ginger.

Transfer the golden milk into cups and garnish with a dash of black pepper.

Pineapple Ginger Lemonade

Ingredients:

- One cup of raw Pineapple pieces
- 1/4 cup of freshly extracted lemon juice *(about two to three lemons)*
- 2–3 teaspoons of freshly grated ginger
- Four cups of water
- 1/4 cup sugar or honey, depending on taste
- Cubes of ice
- Slices of lemon and wedges of pineapple *(optional)*
- Add optional mint leaves *as a garnish*.

Instruction:

Grated ginger, water, freshly squeezed lemon juice and fresh pineapple chunks should all be combined in a blender.

Process till smooth.

To get rid of any pulp or fibres from the pineapple and ginger, strain the mixture into a pitcher using a fine-mesh strainer.

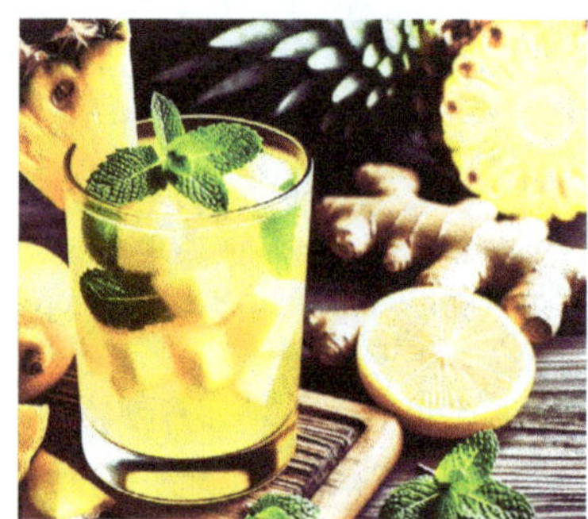

Add the sugar or honey and stir until fully dissolved. *If necessary,* taste and adjust the sweetness.

Let the lemonade cool in the fridge for a minimum of half an hour or until it becomes icy.

Pour the pineapple ginger lemonade into glasses with ice cubes.

If preferred, garnish with mint leaves, pineapple wedges and lemon slices. *Before pouring* - Stir and then serve your cool Pineapple Ginger Lemonade.

Kiwi and Kale Smoothie

Ingredients:

- Peel and cut into two ripe kiwis
- One cup of finely chopped *(stem-free)* kale leaves
- One ripe banana, cut into slices and peeled
- Half a cup of plain Greek yoghurt *(or a vegan option, a dairy-free substitute)*
- 1/2 cup almond milk, unsweetened *(or any other kind of milk)*
- One tablespoon of maple syrup or honey *(optional; adds sweetness)*
- **(Optional, for a cooler smoothie)** Ice cubes

Instruction:

Thoroughly wash the kale leaves and cut off the stiff stems.

After peeling, cut the banana and kiwis into smaller pieces.

Put the banana, Greek yoghurt, almond milk, chopped kale, sliced kiwi and honey or maple syrup *(if using)* in a blender.

If you want your smoothie cooler, feel free to add a few ice cubes.

Blend for 1 to 2 minutes on high speed, scraping down the sides of the blender as needed, until the mixture is smooth and creamy.

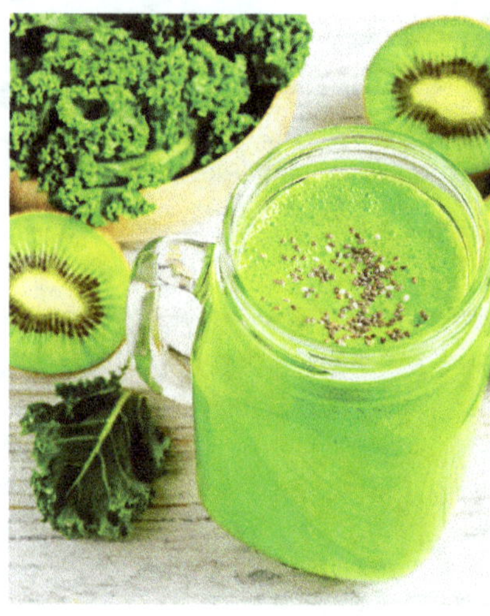

After tasting the smoothie, add additional honey, maple syrup or almond milk *if necessary* to modify the sweetness or consistency.

When the smoothie is smooth, serve it right away by pouring it into glasses.

To fit your tastes and dietary requirements, feel free to alter it by adding more fruits or ingredients like spinach, chia seeds or protein powder.

Carrot Orange Ginger Juice

Ingredients:

- 4 big carrots, cleaned and de-seeding

- One-inch chunk of peeled Ginger
- 2 oranges, both peeled and segmented
- Cubes of ice *(optional)*

Instruction:

To make the carrots fit down the juicer chute, wash, peel and cut them into smaller pieces.

After peeling, cut the oranges into pieces.

Slice the ginger into tiny pieces after peeling it.

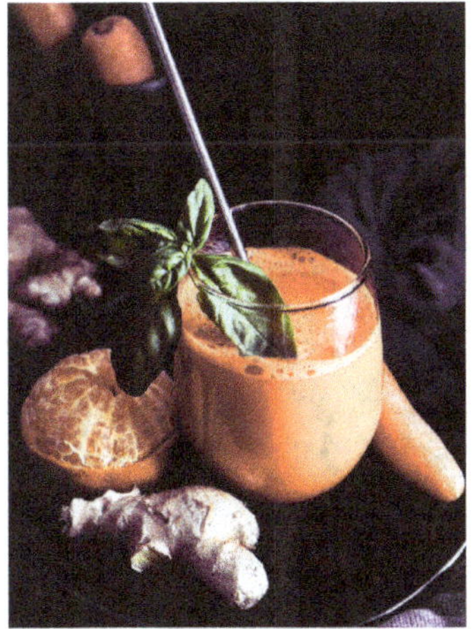

Feed the oranges, ginger and carrots into the juicer in turn.

After juicing all the ingredients, stir the juice to blend the flavours.

Pour the juice into a glass with ice cubes *if you'd like,* and serve.

You may change the amounts of each ingredient to suit your own tastes. For even more flavour diversity, you may also add a sprinkle of cinnamon or a splash of lemon juice.

Chia Seed Lemonade

The sharpness of lemon and the nutritional advantages of chia seeds come together in a delicious and healthful drink called chia seed lemonade.

Ingredients:

- Four glasses of water
- one-fourth cup chia seeds
- 1/2 cup of recently extracted lemon juice, made from around 3–4 lemons.
- 1/4 cup of maple syrup or honey *(adjust to taste)*
- Cubes of ice *(optional)*
- Slices of lemon are **optional** as a garnish.
- **Add optional** mint leaves as a garnish.

Instruction:

Put the chia seeds and water in a big pitcher and mix well to blend.

Stir the chia seeds periodically while letting them soak in the water for 10 to 15 minutes. *This enables the chia seeds to expand and take on the consistency of gel.*

Pour the freshly squeezed lemon juice into the pitcher once the chia seeds have soaked and thickened.

To sweeten the lemonade, stir in honey or maple syrup, adjusting the quantity to suit your taste.

If you want your flavour to be more tart, you may also add more lemon juice.

To cool the lemonade, you may either add ice cubes to the pitcher or refrigerate it for about 1 hour before serving.

Give the lemonade one more swirl to make sure the chia seeds are dispersed evenly. *If preferred,* garnish the glasses of chia seed lemonade with mint leaves and lemon slices.

Modify the lemonade's sweetness and sharpness to suit your tastes. For a different take, try experimenting with additional flavours like fresh berries or herbs like basil.

You can also get the -

Post - Liver Transplant Diet Guide and Cookbook

Which includes steps and tips to home recovery.